304

The Risk Takers

Hugh McLeave

The Risk Takers

HOLT, RINEHART AND WINSTON

New York / Chicago / San Francisco

85617-0113
Printed in the United States of America

Contents

Illustrations

ILLUSTRATIONS

Introduction

THE surgeon had triumphed over everything else. The brain, the eyes, the lungs, the stomach, the limbs—no part of the body was a stranger to his knife. Except the heart. Wrapped in mystery and mysticism throughout twenty centuries, this organ had defied the surgeon and his scalpel and stood challenging him as the last anatomical frontier.

This final frontier of surgery is no more. Every day in hospitals all over the world surgeons are repairing heart defects with much the same ease as they take out an appendix. In some of these operations the heart is isolated from the rest of the body and stopped while its defects are made good; in others the surgeon may virtually switch off life like a light and then restore it again.

Though most of these gains have been made since the Second World War, behind them lies the story of half a century of surgical daring, of triumph mixed with tragedy, of life-and-death risk. The heart did not yield tamely, and the surgeon who tampered with it knew only too well that he could expect no second chance if he failed.

Before the day of the heart-lung machine the surgeon who used a scalpel on the heart took a grave risk. The heart specialist sent his cases to the operating theatre only when he had unavailingly tried everything else and proved in the process how hopeless were their chances. To operate on these last-ditch cases, the surgeon needed cool nerve, a steady hand, faith in himself and a fine disregard for the stares of his colleagues if the mortality rate ran high. Surgeons are human; death is inhuman. Not only did mistakes have to be explained to fellow-surgeons and the boards of governors of hospitals—there were relatives to face. Some surgeons found it difficult to accept the death-rate in early heart techniques, and gave up. But always someone came along willing to take heart surgery that stage further; if necessary, to gamble his reputation doing it.

Sharing the credit for many of the surgical triumphs were the patients—both those who died and those who lived to achieve anonymous though historical mention in the annals of surgery. Heart diseases leave the patient with the grim choice between the short, crippled existence and surgery which will prolong his life. But the man who operated would be the first to pay tribute to the courage and trust of patients who, knowing the odds against success and survival, still put their lives in the hands of the surgeon.

Today, an operation to repair a hole in the heart or to fix its valves has become commonplace; but it took two thousand years for surgery to travel thus far. Today, the surgeon stops and starts the heart while he uses an artificial pump and lungs in its place; but forty years of thinking and planning went into those robots.

We owe the modern wonders of heart surgery to a few dedicated men who laid their foundations brick by brick, men who often ran personal as well as professional risks to push forward into the unknown country of surgery and translate what passed for miracles into workaday routine.

Ironically, the methods and the machines which these pioneers created seem to have overshadowed the men who inspired them. The open-heart operation, the stopped-heart technique, deep-freeze surgery—these and other medical marvels have been accepted by doctors and the public alike, while we forget that their ground work was won slowly and painstakingly over half a century in which success and failure played alternate parts. I hope this book will do something to put the credit where it belongs—with the risk takers.

I

A Road 2,400 Years Long

THE FIGURE lay on the pavement beside the cobbled street oblivious of the raw chill of the autumn night. Past this inert human bundle walked scores of people, and those who noticed, shrugged, probably dismissing it as yet another drunk, and hurried on to the next flickering patch of gaslight illuminating the back streets of Frankfurt.

For fully three hours the man lay where he had fallen before he began to twitch back into consciousness. Painfully he dragged himself to his feet and then groped his way along the pavement towards one of the main streets. Three hundred steps he lurched before sagging once again to the ground beside the street, almost deserted at that hour of the morning.

Soon, several people gathered round the limp figure and gave a harder look when the man did not stir or respond to their questions. The blood on the pavement caught their attention first. Then the deathly face of a young man, in his twenties, with his shirt sodden from a running wound in his chest. When the police took him to the Frankfurt City Hospital, the night staff tut-tutted with the compassion that they show to someone who has gone beyond medical attention.

By then, fragments of the story had begun to emerge. The man's name was Wilhelm Justus; he was twenty-two, an apprentice gardener, though until a few days before he had been in the German Army. Shortly before midnight, Justus had been seen, drunk, in a waterfront café by the River Main and had become involved in a brawl. The police had picked up the kitchen knife which had inflicted the wound, had followed the trail of blood two hundred yards long and came across Justus at 3 a.m.

At the hospital, Dr. Siegel, the house surgeon, looked at the deep wound between the fourth and the fifth ribs then took a thin probe and carefully inserted it along the line of the stab. "In the heart . . . we can do nothing much for him . . . they never recover." As a mere formality they jotted down the case notes, made Justus comfortable with a shot of morphine and placed an ice-pack over the wound. The date they inked in as the eighth of September, 1896. But Dr. Siegel left the police in no doubt that before midnight that day, or perhaps the next, they would have a murder case on their hands.

The young German soldier manifested all the classical signs of a severe heart wound. His face and hands lay grey on the bed, his eyes, the pupils narrowed, had sunk into his head and he shivered and sweated alternately. His breath came in gasps and his pulse under the hospital physician's fingers, fluttered weakly.

But the duty doctor and the nurses were wrong when they gave him a few hours. Somehow he held on until the next day and the night staff marked his chart: "To see Dr. Rehn."

Dr. Ludwig Rehn, Head of the Surgical Department of the City Hospital, was a man whose name had spread beyond the German provincial town through his work on diseases of the throat and chest wounds and the new operation for appendicitis.

The surgeon came to look at the dying man in the early evening of the 9th of September. A stocky, strong figure of 47, his close-cropped brown hair flecked with grey, Rehn still carried himself like the Hussar he had been in the Franco-Prussian war twenty-six years before. He wore the full-faced pointed beard which his Kaiser had popularized.

Carefully, he went over the chart and then examined the

patient. The knife had entered the chest at the fourth rib space and seemed to have penetrated two or three inches. Rehn considered it might have gone through the pericardium, the sac surrounding the main muscle of the heart, and possibly even pierced one of the chambers. The man had lost a great deal of blood and the shocked pallor of the previous night still lay on his face. Though it was then almost seven-thirty in the evening Rehn told the staff to prepare the young man for operation.

In those days a heart operation amounted in itself to a death sentence. The leaders of surgery, practical men who would amputate a leg in two minutes flat, or hustle through a major stomach operation, still looked at the heart with a mixture of dread and superstitious awe. Was it not the seat of the emotions? Was it not the crowning jewel in God's handiwork? Did it not have such precise mechanism to regulate its movements that the slightest touch with the knife would stop it like a watch with a broken mainspring? It was the great surgical untouchable.

Surgeons had tried to make several daring assaults on the heart; to remove bullets or shrapnel; to staunch blood flowing from open wounds; to patch up tears in the heart sac and beyond. All had failed.

Rehn had seen many of those wounds during his service in France. Like his colleagues, he had observed they meant one thing: Death. With his 22-year old patient he would have won the backing of eminent authority had he decided to leave ill alone and watch him die. The great Theodor Billroth, doyen of Viennese surgeons, had waggled his spade beard when he heard idle talk of heart surgery and pronounced: "The surgeon who attempts to operate on the heart cannot wish to preserve the respect of his colleagues."

In England, too, such surgery had short shrift. Only that year, a few months before Rehn faced his dilemma, the influential Stephen Paget had written: "Surgery of the heart has

probably reached the limits set by Nature to all surgery; no
new methods, no new discovery, can overcome the natural
defects that attend a wound of the heart." The views of
these two oracles found faithful echoes throughout the upper
stratum of the profession.

To this Rehn gave a simple answer: "If we see a case which
may be saved only by operation then it is our duty to operate."

The Frankfurt surgeon had the luck to find a man who had
survived more than twenty-four hours with a deep stab wound
in the heart. Transfusion was then unknown. Anaesthetics and
asepsis, the pillars of modern surgery, demanded more art than
science in the physician of those days and more stamina than
most in the patient.

Stamina, the young man had. The ether, dropped on a gauze
mask, made little difference to his weak pulse.

When Rehn looked at him on the table there were already
signs that the sac enclosing the heart had distended; the heart
itself felt larger by more than an inch when the surgeon tapped
the chest to explore.

Rehn thought for a moment, then, with his scalpel made a
seven-inch incision between the fourth and fifth rib, along the
line of the patient's nipple. Drawing back a flap of flesh he
exposed the fifth rib. This he divided with bone scissors and
bent it inwards to expose the beating, pulsating heart sac. He
opened this and saw at a glance that blood from the inner heart
wound had drained into the sac threatening to choke the heart
action.

To relieve the heart he snipped a bigger cut in the sac to drain
off the blood. Behind the incision he saw the four chambers of
the heart. In the right, lower chamber a wound about one inch
long appeared and from this most of the blood was flowing.

Now came the moment of truth. He still had to grope for
the wound and draw it together with silk stitches. Suturing
holes in a throbbing heart had defied many of his contem-

poraries. Rehn reached with his powerful fingers into the cavity he had made and held the palpitating muscle of the heart in one hand while he carefully drew two loops of silk through the knife tear. A third stitch he placed in the pericardium and drew the heart and its protective sac together. At this the organ protested, stopped beating for a moment . . . and then resumed its rhythm.

For the first time a surgeon had held a human heart in his hands. To the assistants and the nurses crowded into the spartan, white-walled operating theatre it seemed that Rehn had mastered the most awesome organ in the body, that the heart had grown stronger.

With dark-red blood no longer welling out of the wound, the rest became easy. The surgeon watched his staff swab out the heart sac and the pleura, then he closed the wound after ensuring it would drain through the tube he inserted.

Only when the operation was over did the surgeon discover that his patient had been discharged from the German army a few days before—with serious heart trouble!

Rehn was the first to admit that he had been lucky with his patient. Paradoxically, the loss of blood had helped him to survive. By weakening the heart beat it allowed less blood to leak through the open wound which thus had time to form a sealing clot. The cold of the night, too, helped the blood round the wound to congeal more readily. And the slow pulse of the heart gave the surgeon fewer problems in placing his sutures.

But all these things considered, the ninth of September, 1896 was a historic day in the history of heart surgery; the day when surgeons ceased to regard the heart as a mystic organ, as something sacrosanct which at a touch of the scalpel would stop never to start again.

In fourteen days Rehn's young patient was walking around the wards of the hospital. A few days later Rehn described his case in dry, academic terms to the Frankfurt Medical Society. But the paper, no more than 400 words long, brought him letters and invitations from his colleagues all over the world and became a model for aspiring heart surgeons.

They wanted to hear Rehn: they asked, also, to see the man who was walking around with three stitches in his heart. So Rehn and his young patient went next year to the International Surgical Congress in Berlin where Rehn demonstrated his technique. And, before hundreds of surgeons from all over the world the young man peeled off his jacket and shirt. They crowded round him to see the hollow in his left side where the surgeon had resected his ribs. And the heart, as strong as it had ever been, pulsing and bounding beneath the chest wall.

One of Rehn's colleagues, Dr. B. F. Sherman, said at the time: "The road to the heart is only two or three centimetres in a direct line, but it had taken surgery nearly 2,400 years to travel it." Sir Russel Brock, the British pioneer who was one of the first to operate inside one of the main heart chambers, made this comment: "Rehn's epoch-making operation demonstrated conclusively that the heart of Man was, in some measure at any rate, tolerant of interference."

Much of the supernatural prejudice which surrounded the heart had been chipped away that autumn day in Frankfurt. Rehn kept a tally of his type of case and noted no fewer than 124 in the next ten years. By then, daring individuals like Ferdinand Sauerbruch were carrying on the campaign to bring the heart under the domination of the knife.

The tussle on what some surgeons called "the last anatomical frontier" amounted to no more than a series of skirmishes around the sheath of the heart and its perimeter of tough inner muscle. Bullets, shrapnel and splinters were prised free and the wounds sutured, though the death rate remained high.

But, with the new enlightenment, surgeons now dared to

make open forays on the heart. A few years after Rehn's success, Sauerbruch, who had made an international reputation as a chest surgeon, attempted to "dry out" the heart by tying off its main veins and arteries. He found he could starve the heart for a minute at the time. Several surgeons had talked about reviving the heart when it stopped during an operation; a few had tried and failed. Then, in 1901 came the announcement that Norwegian surgeon Kristian Igelsrud had taken the stopped heart of a 43-year-old woman in his hand and pumped it until it beat of its own accord.

More important than the minor successes was the changed outlook. It might even be possible to treat some heart diseases with surgery, some surgeons thought. In the post-mortem rooms they saw death as a consequence of diseased or defective heart valves, of congenital tragedies. Could we not correct these conditions on the operating table? The more venturesome surgeons were willing to try; the physicians, cautious and dubious, did not mind their colleagues on the other side of the fence playing about with the outside of the heart. But the inside: NEVER.

This clash between surgeon and physician stopped the clock for many years on heart surgery. For the surgeon depended on his colleague for patients, and to say that someone was a candidate for heart surgery brought a look of cool scepticism from the physician and firm shake of the head. So heart surgery, through the First World War and for many years afterwards, stayed a matter of life and death, a question of stab and bullet wounds, of cases that the physicians had renounced as hopeless.

To saddle the physicians with all of the blame would be less than just. To them the heart still ranked as the most vital organ in the body, one with which no one could tamper with impunity. Many of them shared the Mediaeval belief, endorsed by William Harvey, who discovered the circulation, that the blood flowing through the heart was the seat of the soul.

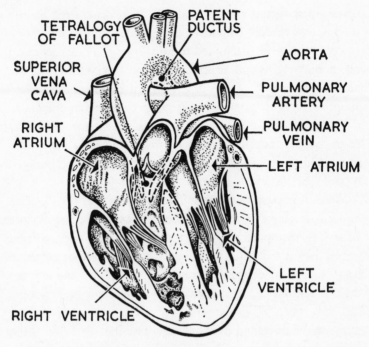

TETRALOGY OF FALLOT

PATENT DUCTUS

SUPERIOR VENA CAVA

AORTA

PULMONARY ARTERY

RIGHT ATRIUM

PULMONARY VEIN

LEFT ATRIUM

LEFT VENTRICLE

RIGHT VENTRICLE

Some major heart defects: the patent ductus, or short-circuit between the main and the lung arteries; the group of deformities shown in the centre of the heart is known as the Tetralogy of Fallot

What is this organ which inspired so much respect in the physician and surgeon? The heart is essentially a pump; though given the task of designing such a pump the engineer would toss back the answer in one word: Impossible. For in the space of not more than six inches by four by three, with a weight of no more than twelve ounces, the heart has to fulfil a powerful and versatile function. At rest it pumps an average of about a gallon of blood a minute, but under pressure it can raise this to nine gallons a minute.

It reacts instantly to every body strain like an engine to the accelerator. But it has no gears to help take the strain. This muscular dynamo has to beat two thousand five hundred million times during the average life span. And normally the

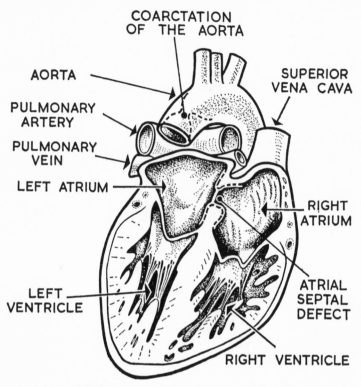

COARCTATION
OF THE AORTA

AORTA

SUPERIOR
VENA CAVA

PULMONARY
ARTERY

PULMONARY
VEIN

LEFT ATRIUM

RIGHT
ATRIUM

LEFT
VENTRICLE

ATRIAL
SEPTAL
DEFECT

RIGHT VENTRICLE

Further heart defects: the constriction of the aorta, or main outlet artery, and
atrial septal defect, or hole between the upper chambers

heart needs no repairs and maintenance that it cannot do while
you sleep. Even then, with the heart idling, it still drives blood
round the body at seventy-five gallons an hour.

The heart is indeed awesome. If it falters, the body soon feels
the consequences. If it fails for three seconds the lack of blood
and oxygen to the brain cuts out consciousness. And, three
minutes after this organ ceases to pump blood to the brain, the
higher nerve cells there begin to perish beyond the recall of any
physician.

The heart itself lies in its smooth, oily sheath, the pericardium, against which its own slippery outer walls beat. The
main structure is a double pump, the halves resembling each

other. At the top the two antechambers, or atria,—they used
to be called auricles, or "little ears" because of their shape—
collect blood from the veins and the lungs. They then force
this blood through valves to the ventricles, the main pumping
chambers, which drive it out to the main arteries and to the
lungs.

The heart beats with impressive discipline. First the atria
which have filled with spent blood from the veins and fresh
blood from the lungs contract to squeeze their contents into the
ventricles. The top chambers then relax as the more powerful

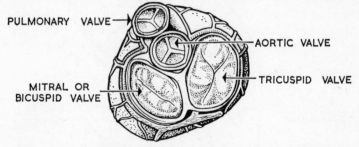

This sectional drawing indicates the four heart valves, the leaves of which may
be fused together to prevent free blood flow. Or the valves may fail to close
properly and thus work incompetently.

ventricles contract. The right chamber thrusts the blood
through the pulmonary artery round the lungs; the left compartment forces it through the aorta, the blood main serving
the whole body.

The immense power of the organ comes from spiral bands
of muscle surrounding the ventricles. These muscles snap into
compression against the thick walls of the two chambers and
literally wring the blood out through the arteries. It is their
rebound from this fierce contraction phase that pulls the blood
through from the two top reservoir chambers.

To prevent blood flowing back into the reservoirs or from
the arteries, the heart has four valves. Incidentally, the sounds
that we can pick up in major arteries are shock waves from
the biggest of these valves as they snap shut.

How does the heart maintain its rhythm? At one time doctors believed that the "metronome" of the heart consisted of nerve cells and fibres in the muscles. Nowadays, the heart pacemaker is known to lie behind the right atrium as a specialized knot of muscle tissue which generates weak electric shocks. These run through the heart like a flame through gunpowder, triggering off first the contraction of the atria and, a split second later, the lower chambers.

In the days before and after the First World War, physicians and surgeons had only a vague understanding of the action of the heart. A physician needed a trained ear and more than ordinary talent to make sense of the faulty rhythms and the "murmurs" on which he eavesdropped with his stethoscope; the art of X-raying the heart to confirm enlargement of its chambers still had far to go. So it was in the dissecting room that most of the detective work took place—when the heart had long since ceased to beat.

One factor became clear: much of the trouble lay with the heart valves. These were often found to be diseased or thickened so that they did not close properly, or perhaps closed too much. Some of these cases had been "cardiac cripples" from birth; in most, valvular disease had been a legacy of rheumatic fever or some infective disease which had attacked the valves, scarring them and weakening their action.

Whatever the cause, hundreds of cases appeared in clinics and hospitals where doctors could only prescribe stimulants, a few sympathetic words and the admonition to take things easy. Nothing could be done.

A few surgeons thought otherwise. In the early twenties two groups of American surgeons began to wonder if they could not relieve some valvular diseases. They had seen in the dissecting room that much of the heart trouble centred around the mitral valve, so-called because its cusps are shaped like a Bishop's mitre. This large two-leaved valve lies between the

upper and lower chambers on the left side of the heart, opens
to admit blood from the atrium to the ventricle, and then snaps
shut to prevent a return of blood and loss of pumping pressure
when the powerful ventricle contracts.

The American surgeons knew from earlier work that sometimes the valve was incompetent—the cusps did not close to
seal the opening. But the other classical condition interested
them much more, where the segments of the mitral valve had
stuck together, narrowing the gap and cutting the flow of
blood into the main pumping chamber. Would it be possible to
get at the valve and break the seal with a knife?

The Americans were daring enough to pierce the lower
left chamber with a tiny double-edged scalpel and feel blindly
for the valve. Even with the heart bounding irregularly in their
hands they claimed some success with the method. From these
attempts it became obvious that surgery had something to
offer: but just as evident were the great risks which this hit-
and-miss surgery involved.

In Britain a few like-minded men had similar ideas for
operating on the heart valves.

2

Six Months to Live

FOR YEARS Henry Souttar had considered operating on the heart. Against the main current of medical opinion he had held that it might even be possible to enter the heart itself and lever apart the petals of blocked valves to permit the human pump to work properly.

Like many surgeons, Souttar had an inventive mind. In 1920 he took a second look at one of the instruments of surgery as old as the knife itself—the needle. Surgeons still used their refinement of the curved sailmaker's needle threading their silk through the eye. Souttar considered that with catgut you could fashion the blunt end of the needle into a socket for the gut. He had a piece of silver drawn into the shape of a bootlace tag, fitted the gut into it and crimped the end. Now, operating theatres all over the world use Souttar's Eyeless Needle.

At 48 years of age, greying and with years of surgery in London, all over the world and on the battlefields of Belgium behind him, Souttar was working as consultant surgeon to the London Hospital. The biggest hospital in the country brought him more than enough work. But between cases, the tall, athletic figure could be seen bending over some experiment in the dissecting room.

"I began with animals," he said. "I believed at first that it might be feasible to make artificial valves out of metal and rubber to replace incompetent or stenosed valves. But, after some time, I gave it up. It seemed we could not do as well as Nature."

He had read of the American work, had studied, too, the results of post-mortem research on heart valves by English surgeons like Strickland Goodall and Lambert Rogers. Man-made valves were out; but could not a skilled surgeon do something for the crippled ones that condemned patients to a fragile and breathless life?

Souttar thought he knew the answer to this question, and began by himself to examine the valves of the heart in the post-mortem room. He found he could easily divide joined valve petals, either by pushing his finger through them or by splitting them with a small, double-edged scalpel. If he could clear the stenosis on a dead heart, why not on a live one?

One grave snag faced him—in the shape of an eminent Scots physician to whom virtually the whole of the medical profession deferred on questions of heart disease. Sir James Mackenzie, born in the old Scottish capital of Scone, had become the "baron" of the London Hospital and was, in the early 'twenties, at the pinnacle of a long and distinguished career. Brilliant, hard-headed but testy, Sir James, the King's Physician, had written the only books that mattered to British doctors on heart disease. His West End consulting rooms filled with all types of society; to see the stern figure in a high wing collar, with a King Edward the Seventh beard, doctors and students crammed his lecture room at the London Hospital.

When Souttar ventured to express himself about the possibility of operating on the heart valves his colleagues gave him a glassy-eyed stare and changed the topic. Carried to the ear of Sir James, the surgeon's ideas met a derisive and dour resistance. "Operations on the valves—indeed," snorted Sir James. "The only heart disease I know of is that of the muscle. And no operation that I've heard of will correct this."

Undismayed, Souttar continued his experiments—and quietly he waited for the right patient. "It was two years," he recalled, "before anyone referred such a patient to me."

Unknown to the surgeon there was such a patient in the hospital while he was doing penance in the post-mortem room. She was a thin waif of a girl who lived in the poor East End district of Whitechapel, near the old, sprawling hospital. And she bore the classical signs of mitral stenosis, the very condition on which Souttar had done most of his work.

Lily Hine had been brought to the London Hospital by her parents when they noticed that the slightest effort left her exhausted and gasping for breath. A dark, bright-eyed child, Lily had made frequent appearances at the hospital from 1921 onwards, often coming in for weeks to rest and restore the dregs of strength which her weak heart had left her.

Again and again, her doctors found her symptoms recurring, each time worse than the last. A bright flush lay over her pretty, pale face; her pulse more often than not beat twice as fast as it should; the pulsation even fluttered noticeably across her chest when she breathed in quick short gasps.

More disquieting were the sounds picked up by the stethoscope. From the left side of the heart came a long, rumbling "murmur" as the main pumping chamber tensed; when it relaxed another soft, blowing sound superseded the first. Just as the trained mechanic will catch and diagnose the blowing noise of an engine gasket, so the doctors concluded that these heart echoes could mean only one thing: the mitral valve was so badly stuck that it jeopardized the girl's life.

Souttar met the young Cockney girl first in March, 1925, when she was admitted with a rasping cough, severe breathlessness and pain throughout her limbs. To steady the heart they had given her digitalis: for the pain, aspirin. The drugs brought little improvement.

The surgeon saw the heart specialist who was dealing with the case. "How long do you think she has to live?" he asked.

The specialist, Dr. T. B. Layton, replied: "At the very most six months. If you feel you can do anything, then go ahead and try."

The girl's family were consulted and told that such an operation had never before been performed. They agreed that, if the operation might do the child some good, the surgeon could go ahead. Lily, herself, had grown to trust the soft-spoken surgeon and willingly consented when he put it to her.

For Souttar and his staff the risks were obvious. Sir James Mackenzie had died at the beginning of the year but his presence still brooded over the hospital and further afield. Then, as now, the surgeon and anaesthetist who met with failure and death in the operating theatre, had to face the British coroner, a formidable figure with the power to rebuke and reprimand anyone who he thought had risked the life of a patient unnecessarily. "Natural Causes" on the death certificate of a patient who might have been saved by a new operation was one thing; a mistake on the operating table could leave a permanent scar on the reputation of the surgeon and his anaesthetist.

"We might have considered those consequences, but it became more important to us to try to give our patient a second chance," said the surgeon.

The other man who gambled his reputation was the anaesthetist, Dr. John Challis. This slight, self-effacing character was judged to be one of the finest "gas men" in the country at that time. Challis had none of the imposing battery of anaesthetics and equipment which his modern counterpart can command—only ether and chloroform.

In those days anaesthetics caused as many deaths as surgery itself. To give a relatively crude anaesthetic to a girl with a weak heart when the climate of opinion was hostile needed a cool head, dexterity and courage. "When I look back on the situation, I think John Challis did a very brave thing," said Souttar.

The operation, set for May 6th, necessitated careful planning. Souttar, clever as a draftsman, sketched a plan for his surgery, and devised a highly ingenious method of entering the heart without risking massive blood loss.

Lily went quietly under the anaesthetic and Challis slipped the tube which had been invented by his colleague, Ivan Magill, into the windpipe to keep feeding her his ether-chloroform mixture. Souttar took a scalpel and made a long C-shaped cut all the way round the heart and then resected the ribs to expose the rapid, pulsing heart under its protective sac.

A nod from Challis, watching the girl's condition, told them they had to stop. The heart beat had soared to 150 in those few minutes—twice the normal pace. For five long minutes they waited until the pulse slowed and the rhythm steadied.

The surgeon then opened the pericardium with a three-inch incision and saw the top of the left, upper chamber protrude. Meticulously, he placed three stitches through this part of the atrium and drew it forward—but this again sent the pulse up to a dangerous level. Challis injected a drug to steady the heart —but it meant another ten minutes of waiting until the pulse had dropped to 120—still 50 above the normal beat.

Now came the crucial stage. As the heart grew stronger, Souttar drew forward the appendage of the atrium and clamped it across the base. With the clamp sealing the end of the chamber he made a half-inch incision —just wide enough to push his forefinger through into the heart.

He then thrust his forefinger through this hole as though he were drawing on the tight finger of a glove. Immediately the clamp was withdrawn, the surgeon felt the back pressure of blood from the main pumping chamber as it contracted. More eloquently than any diagnosis, this told him that the mitral valve was not working properly.

The stay stitches held the muscle of the heart tight against his forefinger as he explored beyond the mitral valve to the "heart strings" which tie it to the main chamber and prevent the blood pressure pushing it back into the atrium. With each beat the surgeon could feel the valve leaves opening and closing slightly. They had not fused as much as the diagnosis had indicated.

Souttar later wrote in the *British Medical Journal*: "The finger was kept in the auricle for perhaps two minutes, and during that time, so long as it remained in the auricle, it appeared to produce no effect upon the heart beat or the pulse.

"The moment, however, that it passed into the orifice of the mitral valve, the blood pressure fell to zero, although even then no change in the cardiac rhythm could be detected. The blood stream was simply cut off by the finger which presumably just fitted the stenosed orifice."

Before the operation, Souttar had decided to section the valve with a knife, but since he found little thickening, he satisfied himself by breaking down the adhesions with his forefinger.

They had accomplished what they had intended. Now it became merely a matter of retracing their steps. But, when the real danger had passed, they nearly lost the patient.

As Souttar gently withdrew his finger from the auricle, the silk which should have closed the incision snapped. Blood spurted from the upper chamber and the girl's blood pressure sagged dangerously. Worse still, the appendage through which the heart had been entered, slid back into the pericardium.

Quickly, the surgeon pressed the leaking atrium against the heart wall to staunch the blood flow while one of his assistants deftly tied off the hole. An audible gasp of relief ran round the theatre as the blood pressure began to climb again and the surgeon could close the chest. The clock showed that Souttar's operation had taken only sixty minutes which is quick, even by present-day standards.

Later the surgeon wrote in the *British Medical Journal*: "Except at the moment when the suture cut out, her condition had never caused the slightest anxiety, and even then there was only a momentary drop in the blood pressure."

He added a few comments which, to his sceptical colleagues, must have sounded the height of medical heresy.

"There can," he said, "be no more fascinating problem in surgery than the relief of pathological conditions of the valves of the heart. We are, however, of the opinion that these conditions again are purely mechanical, and that, apart from them, the heart is as amenable to surgical treatment as any other organ. Incisions can be made in its chambers, portions of its structure can be excised and internal manipulations carried out without the slightest interference with its action, and there is ample evidence that wounds of the heart heal as readily as those in any other region."

As though to confirm his words, Lily Hine showed a marked improvement from the day of the operation. She said so herself. No longer did she pay for the slightest movement with a livid complexion and choking breathlessness. "Every so often she would come into the hospital to let us have a look at her. I think we gave her another five years of life, and it was a completely different condition that killed her—a brain clot."

His daring tussle with the heart won Souttar few friends, and no honours. In general the profession pooh-poohed his remarks on heart operations; the spectre of Sir James Mackenzie still stalked his own and other hospitals; and, though privately congratulated by his close colleagues on the skill and ingenuity of the operation, no physician and surgeon attempted to emulate his technique. The heart patients still came in their hundreds, most of them suffering from mitral stenosis, Lily Hine's disease. But they went out through the same hospital door as in they came. Henry Souttar never had the chance to follow up his one success. No one ever sent him another case of mitral valve disease.

Not until 1949, when he was 74 and had added a great many

honours to his name, did the surgeon receive a knighthood. By then surgeons in England and America were performing his operation as a routine. American surgeons Charles P. Bailey of Philadelphia, and Dwight E. Harken, of Harvard medical school, had heard of a British operation before they made their attempt in 1948. There, in the yellowing files of the *British Medical Journal*, they read Souttar's eloquently descriptive account of the first successful surgical invasion of the heart. And they wondered that the British medical profession had been so slow to take up the challenge where Souttar left off. For only in the post-war years did a few English surgeons revive their interest in heart surgery. Almost a whole generation of silence had fallen over the field, and it was some time before British cardiac surgeons could point with some pride to the fact that they had caught up with the Americans.

When I met him at the age of 86, Sir Henry Souttar showed no resentment, only regret that so many cases which might have been helped or even cured had been given up. He left me with this wry and ironical comment. "I am," he said, "the only surgeon in the world who operated on the heart with no mortality."

The story of the heart moved from Britain to America—and across to Germany where it had begun.

3

The Man who Gambled His Life

YOUNG Dr. Werner Forssmann was rummaging through one of the cupboards in his home when his eye fell on the old veterinary journal. He flicked over the pages and then a print in the book caught his attention. It showed a veterinary surgeon passing a long, slim tube into the vein of a horse to take blood samples. The picture fascinated the 25-year-old German doctor. Could he pass such a hollow tube down a vein into the human heart?

Forssmann was then, in 1929, working at Eberswalde, fifty miles north of Berlin. He discussed his ideas with his colleagues in the small surgical clinic, but they were not impressed. Thrust a tube into the heart! Even if you succeeded, they asked, what good would it do? Privately they thought the stern-faced doctor an eccentric and spoke among themselves of his "circus tricks". Some of them did not doubt he would kill himself or someone else if he tried the experiment.

Patiently, Forssmann explained that passing a catheter tube through the vein into the heart would enable doctors to give emergency drug treatment during operations. He opposed, he said, the present method of injecting drugs straight into the heart because this damaged the coronary vessels and might cause the organ to fail.

His first experiment he made on a dead body. The oiled-rubber catheter slipped effortlessly along the vein and Forssmann pushed it about twenty inches, until he satisfied himself that it had entered the right upper chamber of the heart. The left arm, he observed, seemed the best starting place, for in this way the tube approached the heart in a long, smooth curve.

The next stage would normally have been animal experiments, but Forssmann could not obtain guinea pigs at the small surgical unit. Nor could he attempt such a perilous procedure on anyone else. Could he try it on himself? Use himself as a human guinea pig? Half a dozen times he ventured to insert a tube in his arm before deciding that he needed the help of a colleague. He begged a doctor friend to assist him in the experiment and the man reluctantly agreed.

At the crook of Forssman's elbow they made an incision, cut a main vein and passed a wide-bore needle into it. The colleague slid the oiled rubber tube down the needle and along the vein. Inch by inch it glided up the arm while Forssmann stood impassively, reporting only slight pain, but no real discomfort. His colleague did not share his equanimity. When some sixteen inches of tube had been paid out the other doctor thought that he might kill Forssmann, and refused to go on with the experiment. Reluctantly, both abandoned the attempt.

But Forssmann, determined to complete the sounding of the heart or accept the consequences of failure and the fatal injury that it might cause, decided to go it alone. He waited a week and then, with his scalpel, his needle and catheter he went into the small operating theatre of the clinic. His only assistant was a nurse, who privately thought the young doctor was taking dedication to research much too far, but concluding that someone had to remain on hand in case the experiment led to tragedy, she unwillingly agreed to help.

First, Forssmann injected a local anaesthetic into the crook of his arm and when it turned numb he dissected his own vein and, with difficulty, inserted the needle and catheter tube into it. Slipping the first few inches of the tube inside the vein, the doctor positioned himself behind a continuous X-ray screen. The nurse had a mirror before the screen to allow Forssmann

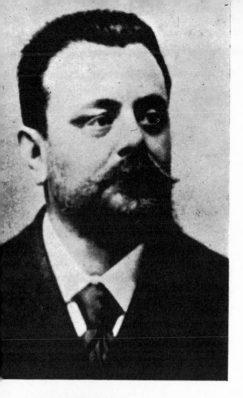

Three pioneers of heart surgery. *Left:* Etienne Fallot, the French physician who first described the four heart defects known as the Tetralogy of Fallot. *Below left:* Ludwig Rehn, the Frankfurt surgeon who first operated successfully on the heart in 1896. Rehn proved that the heart could be repaired by sewing up a deep stab wound. *Below right:* Werner Theodore Otto Forssmann at the age of 25, when he performed a life-or-death experiment on himself by slipping a rubber tube through his left arm vein and into the heart chamber itself.

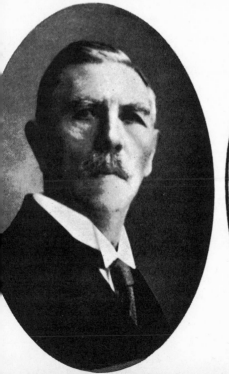

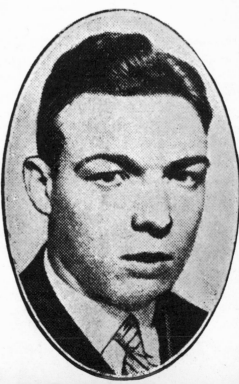

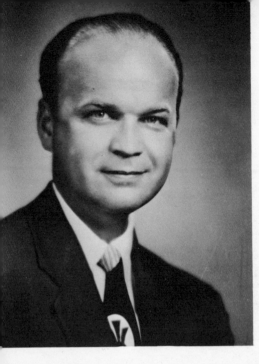

Dr. C. Walton Lillehei, one of the most brilliant of modern heart surgeons. Lillehei and his team at the University of Minnesota have pioneered many techniques for heart surgery, including the first series of open-heart operations for major defects, and have been responsible for many innovations in pacemaking and patching faulty hearts

A view of the team at the University of Minnesota. Dr. Lillehei and his assistant work on a heart defect while theatre staff and technicians monitor the battery of machines around the operating table. In the centre of the background is the Lillehei-De Wall machine, one of the first successful heart-lung robots

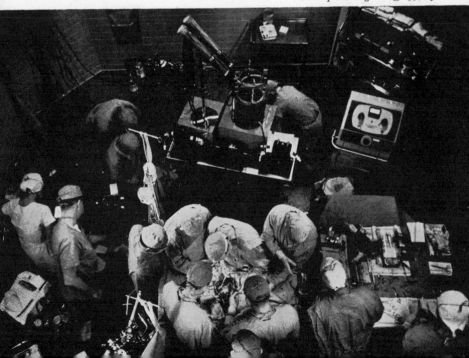

to watch the progress of the tube as it crept up the inside of his arm towards the heart.

Up and up he eased it, until it followed the curve of the armpit and slid towards the heart. As it slid along the vein, he reported to the nurse that he felt a tingling pain in the arm. Then, again, as the tube, like a thick strand of silver thread on the X-ray screen, slid down towards the right atrium of the heart, he announced a burning sensation behind the collar band. Carefully he manipulated the tube towards this receiving chamber—until he saw it enter the pulsating organ. With some satisfaction, he observed that the heart maintained its steady rhythm.

It was done. But would they believe him? The X-ray screen only monitored the tube, but did not fix the image. When he retracted it, there would be nothing but his own description of the experiment. Forsmann then did something which makes even the most iron-clad medical research worker quail.

With the catheter still inside his heart he walked from the operating room, through a long corridor and up two flights of stairs to the radiological department. His arm tingled and grew warm as he moved. But he waited until several X-ray pictures had been taken to show the tube leading from his arm into his heart.

When his paper with two of the X-rays appeared in the *Klinische Wochenschrift*, Forsmann discovered that another German doctor had already succeeded with catheterization. Dr. Fritz Bleichroeder, medical director of a small women's hospital in Berlin, had inserted tubes into the thigh veins of patients. But his studies, done at the turn of the century, had not been published. X-ray equipment in those days failed to record the experiments and Bleichroeder, a modest man, often did not care to publish many of his findings.

Forssmann generously acknowledged his colleague's work, and then began to test the theory which had inspired him to risk his life. He tried to pipe drugs directly into the heart through tubes, but soon gave this up as unsuccessful. He then turned to the possibility of using catheters for diagnosis of heart disease. Here, he foresaw many of the techniques by which doctors not only sound the heart through catheters, but inject drugs into it. "To conclude," he said in the *Klinische Wochenschrift*, "I should like to point out that this method opens up new possibilities for research into the metabolism and the activity of the heart which I am already investigating."

Following the publication of his paper Forssmann received an invitation to join the staff of the famous Charité Hospital in Berlin and work with men like Sauerbruch, the renowned chest surgeon. But the young experimenter stuck it for only a short time. The profession still considered him slightly crankish for having attempted the experiment; they did not forgive him for having succeeded. Disillusioned, he returned to Eberswalde to establish himself in practice as a general physician. He still considered that cardiac catheterization had an important role in diagnosis of heart conditions, and he kept on experimenting with methods of using the tube-in-the-heart technique for X-ray diagnosis, more or less ignored by German surgeons and physicians.

Forssmann found himself thwarted in his efforts to interest the medical profession and finally gave up his experiments. Even his general practice in Eberswalde dwindled, and in the thirties he quit the small German town for Berlin. He became the man who had carried out a foolish and risky manœuvre on himself and published one obscure paper on a dead-end technique which no one could use. For all the medical profession knew or cared Forssmann had sunk without trace. In 1944 he was found to be working in a Berlin hospital. Medicine had been so unkind to him and his family that he decided after the war to forsake the profession. And, for a year, he did, earning his living by felling trees.

But that obscure paper had not lain unread. The first advances in heart surgery revealed the need for more accurate diagnosis of cardiac conditions. Two doctors in the United States of America followed up the clues which Forssman had scattered around. Their work paved the way for some of the surgical advances of the forties and fifties. It brought Forssmann out of obscurity to share the Nobel Prize with the doctors André Cournand and Dickinson W. Richards.

4

Surprise for Sauerbruch

SLOWLY, year by year, the heart was giving up its secrets. Surgeons still paid their respects to it, but no longer as the fragile seat of the emotions or the capricious and mysterious creation which would resist their knives. No, it seemed more lusty and tough than most other organs and had come through many thousands of severe wounds and several encroachments with the scalpel.

But, in general, the surgeon who wanted to make a name for himself left the heart alone during the thirties. He only had to consult the literature to realize that more than a few up-and-coming colleagues had either ruined their reputation or grown disillusioned in their attempts to tame this rebellious organ.

But advances were made—some of them by sheer accident.

A 28-year-old German woman came into the Charité Hospital in Berlin in 1931 to consult the great Ferdinand Sauerbruch. She was ill, breathless, and the pain in her chest suggested to the physicians and the surgeon that she had a cancer either of the food tract or on the lung. X-rays seemed to substantiate this finding, and when Sauerbruch saw them he decided to perform an operation to excise the tumour.

At 55, Sauerbruch was the doyen of German surgeons, a man of international repute with a long history of brilliant surgery behind him. He had conceived the low-pressure chamber which made much early lung surgery possible and the medical profession knew him as a bold and fearless operator.

With his usual audience in the theatre, Sauerbruch opened the woman's chest and laid bare the sac surrounding the heart. Beneath the pericardium lay a lump which pulsated and seemed to have grown on the heart itself. Thinking that it must be a cyst, Sauerbruch decided to attack it from the right side of the body and incised through the fifth rib space into the area of the swelling. What he saw astonished him; it lay the size of a grapefruit, a fierce lump which appeared to have roots in the centre of the heart.

With dozens of pairs of eyes watching, the German surgeon explored the lump with his fingers. It was a cyst. He should drain it. Then cut it out. With a large-bore, hollow needle he punctured the lump and then withdrew the plunger. Nothing came out. Again, he tried, and this time the syringe filled with blood. The whole operating theatre stood still, wondering what they were dealing with.

No one had time to surmise after that. When the surgeon pulled out the needle the second time a thin jet of blood spurted out of the hole and struck him in the face. Instinctively, an assistant handed Sauerbruch the needle and suturing thread in his hand; instinctively, the surgeon grabbed it and began to ply stitches into the edges of the leaking hole. But, attempting to pull the thread tight, it tore through the thin wall of the swelling. This time, a fountain of blood poured out of the wound, and the surgeon realized what he had encountered.

The heart wall had weakened, and ballooned under pressure until it was ready to burst.

To staunch the blood, Sauerbruch thrust first one finger of his left hand into the hole, then the second, until the elastic wall of the heart closed around them. Both his fingers lay in the right, lower chamber of the heart.

In less gifted hands the woman would surely have died. She had lost blood from an already weakened heart. But she lived. Sauerbruch held his fingers in the heart chamber until his assistant clamped off the swelling. Now they knew what they faced. The heart wall had bulged into an aneurysm the size and shape of a toy balloon. When Sauerbruch had gripped and clamped both edges of the aneurysm he cut out the weakened muscle, stitched the edges and closed the chest. The woman lived to be the first successful case of surgery on a heart aneurysm.

In America and England surgeons had begun to operate on the main bundles of muscle around the heart itself. In 1935 Professor Claude Beck corrected a lack of blood supply to the arteries in the muscle by grafting a part of the chest wall into it. Laurence O'Shaughnessy, with some success, grafted part of the abdominal membrane up through the diaphragm into the heart muscle a year later. These two operations, and variations of them, have been adopted by other surgeons.

The modern assault on the heart really began, however, with an operation not on the organ itself but on the main blood lines leading from it to the body. This time, an American girl made surgical history.

She was seven years of age, scrawny and badly nourished when she came into the Children's Hospital in Boston. All her life she had never known good health, for she had been born a heart cripple. When she was three years old, her doctors had found the congenital defect which sent a strong pulsation over her chest and a loud heart murmur.

When her mother brought her to the Children's Hospital she informed the doctors that she could hear a "buzzing noise" when she stood near her daughter. The child herself often told her mother that she felt "there is something wrong in my chest".

The man who examined the girl was one of America's leading chest and heart surgeons. Dr. Robert E. Gross of Harvard Medical School did not have to look hard to diagnose the type of defect he had to deal with. Over the neck he could see a strong pulse flickering. And when he placed his stethoscope over the arteries in the arm and thigh he heard what he described as "pistol shot sounds". The prominent chest veins, the rough "machinery murmur" over the heart, the X-rays, which showed ballooning of the heart—they could mean only one thing: the child was suffering from a large-scale blood leakage from one main heart artery to another.

Patent Ductus Arteriosus this inborn defect was called. Every child is born with a patent, or open, duct between the main artery and the branch line which carries blood from the heart to the lungs. To prevent blood being pumped to the lungs before they begin to function, this channel shunts blood from the pulmonary artery into the main artery. Normally it closes three days after birth, but in some cases this arterial duct stays open.

When the strong left ventricle begins to squeeze high-pressure blood into the main artery some of it by-passes through the defect into the lung artery which works at lower pressure. Damage to the lung can therefore result and children with such deformities often fall victim to bronchitis, tire easily and sometimes suffer from stunted growth. Not only did the deformity condemn children to invalidism; the heart would compensate for the defect only to a certain extent, then rebel and give up. Gross and his colleagues knew that such conditions laid the heart open to infection for which the patient had little resistance.

The girl came into the Children's Hospital on the 17th August, 1938, and for nine days she waited for the operation while surgeons and physicians studied her condition and the seven-foot chest X-ray they had taken.

On the morning of the 26th of August they wheeled her into the theatre. Dr. Gross decided to enter the heart through the left side and made his incision along the third rib space. The surgeon allowed the left lung to collapse, baring the sac which covered the heart and its arteries. This, he slit to expose the main blood trunkline, the aorta, rising in its arch over the top of the heart. Running underneath were the lung arteries which should normally have had no connection with the main artery.

But there, between the aorta and the artery taking spent blood to the lungs, lay the channel through which blood pounded from the strongest pumping chamber. It was wide, about a third of an inch, but only a fifth of an inch long.

The surgeon explored the outside of the open duct with his finger and felt a tremor over the whole of this region of the heart. Gross then listened with a sterile stethoscope and heard the loud blowing of a murmur over the whole organ.

As he wrote in the *Journal of the Medical Association*, "When the stethoscope was placed on the pulmonary artery there was an almost deafening, continuous roar, sounding very much like a large volume of steam escaping in a closed room."

Round the vessel the surgeon drew a thick piece of silk thread and held it there while he and his staff watched the clock for three long minutes to see how the heart and lungs would behave. They were tense minutes. Within the loop of thick silk lay a blood vessel which, if it tore or burst, would spill enough blood in seconds to end any attempts to finish the operation. No one stirred as they watched the heart rise and fall and kept an eye on the anaesthetist for signs of heart or breathing failure.

At the end of three minutes there seemed no impairment of the circulation and Gross decided to tie off the vessel permanently. Dramatically, as soon as the surgeon had tightened and knotted the silk thread round the channel the tremor died away. The girl's lung was expanded again, the chest sewn up — and for the first time a surgeon could claim to have cured an inborn defect of the heart.

The operation had transformed the life of the child. She had no sign of surgical shock, only mild discomfort in the afternoon following it. On the second day she was sitting up, and on the third day walked around the ward. The surgeon noted with satisfaction that the blood pressure had dropped nearly to normal and nothing of the violent pulsations was visible.

For the first time since the great Greek physician, Galen, had described the patent ductus in the second century A.D., medicine had succeeded in curing the condition it caused. Gross was not the first to have tried to close the channel which short-circuited blood into the lungs. His colleague in Boston, Dr. John Streider, had operated on a 22-year-old girl sixteen months before and had partially closed the duct—only to lose his patient from stomach infection five days later. But it was Gross's successs which lent courage and inspiration to surgeons to treat open channels between the main arteries from the heart. There was no scarcity of them. Seventeen out of every hundred cases of congenital heart disease have a patent ductus, and, curiously enough, twice as many girls as boys are born with it. The chances of a child suffering from this defect have been estimated as one in 5,500 live births.

Gross kept in touch with his first patient through the years and was one of the first to congratulate her when she married, and later when she had a child. In the next twenty years he and his staff at Harvard carried out 1,500 cases of patent ductus with negligible mortality.

The dozens of surgeons who carried out the Gross operation realized that this defect was not the only one which would yield to surgery; others hitherto regarded as inoperable might also be corrected.

Gross and his colleagues began to study the more simple of the other heart diseases. At that time the Americans and the Swedes had the field of advanced heart surgery virtually to themselves. In Europe, surgeons were donning battle dress and had neither the time nor the opportunity to carry out anything but emergency work. No doubt they gained experience of heart wounds which cropped up in their thousands, and this eroded away much of the blind awe in which the heart had been held. But outside America and Sweden nothing much was achieved in the war years.

It was in the autumn of 1944 that two people walked into the Sabbatsberg Hospital in Stockholm. One of them, a pale-faced, scrawny schoolboy of 12, went to see Dr. Nylin in the department of medicine; the other, a stout, florid-faced farmer, found his way to the surgical clinic to see its chief, Dr. Clarence Crafoord. To the doctors it seemed almost a fatalistic coincidence; for they had been discussing for months the form of heart condition which crippled both patients. And Crafoord had told Nylin that he thought he could cure it with surgery.

Both the schoolboy and the farmer had a constriction in the aorta, the main artery, just after it left the top of the heart. With the boy it was an inborn defect: with the farmer it had recently developed. The kink in this thick pipe narrowed its bore just as the arch of the aorta curved to supply the blood vessels in the lower part of the body. Not only did the obstruction rob these arteries and veins of blood but it built up a pressure in the arteries which branched off to supply the head and the neck. So the condition—called coarctation of the aorta—needs little medical detection. The upper part of the body has a fierce pulse and high blood pressure; the lower half almost no pulse and low blood pressure. It is three times scarcer than patent ductus.

To Crafoord especially, these patients came like an answer to a prayer. This surgeon, one of the world's greatest, had studied the way in which blockages in the blood circulation affected the brain and the organs of the body. Experiments proved to him that, so long as blood carried oxygen to the brain, no harm resulted if the circulation were arrested in other parts of the body. He then, as he recounted, took the risk of clamping the aorta in patients undergoing operations for patent ductus arteriosus, and confirmed that the main blood channel could be obstructed completely for anything up to twenty-seven minutes—without damage to the patient's internal organs. If he could clamp off the aorta this long, surely this would give time to cut out a part of the vessel and join its ends. His colleague, Nylin, agreed.

The Swedish schoolboy who arrived at the clinic complained to the doctors he felt very weak after slight exertion. The doctors made him exercise on a special staircase, and then took heart readings and blood pressures. Crafoord heard much the same story from the farmer. He had been used, he said, to heavy work around his farm, but about six months before he saw his doctor had found he could no longer work without feeling fatigue and a tightness in his chest.

The Swedish surgeon not only faced the problem of arresting the blood supply long enough to finish the surgery. No one had joined a major artery before, though many doctors had pointed to the hazards which might follow such a procedure. A break in the smooth walls of the artery might dam the blood flow, cause a clot and kill the patient. Crafoord got to work evolving different types of stitching which would make a perfect union. Ingeniously, he found that, by turning up the ends of the cut artery as a tailor would the bottoms of trousers, he could join them without leaving a blood trap in the bore of the artery.

Crafoord did the operations within twelve days of each other and discovered they both had the same wedge-shaped narrowing of the aorta as it bent downwards. He clamped each side of the constriction, cut it away and ran stitches round the ends to join them.

The effect was dramatic. The blood pressure fell in the upper half of the body and rose in the lower. Five months later, the farmer reported he was back at work and the schoolboy had lost his weakness.

Crafoord had hardly made his findings known when Gross,

who had experimented with this operation from 1938, reported success. He and Charles Hufnagel, at their second attempt, cured a kink in the aorta by surgery in July, 1945. Independently, they had come to much the same conclusions as Crafoord about the way in which the ends of the artery ought to be joined. Gross went on to work out methods of replacing the excised sections of artery by preserved arterial grafts when it was impossible to draw the ends together.

Crafoord and Gross did dozens of these operations and quickly they became routine in other countries. The pace of heart surgery was quickening, and before the war ended another fragment of the story had been written by two American doctors who conceived and accomplished one of the most daring and ingenious operations in the history of surgery.

5

The Blue-Baby Operation

ERHAPS the most tragic heart cripples are Blue Babies.
The description conveys only some idea of the fragile
child with livid face and lips who lives out a short and
breathless life. Even the minor pleasures of living go beyond
the strength of these children. Eating can mean exhaustion;
walking becomes a grim step-by-step purgatory; and the
simple act of dressing or undressing leaves them weak.

What could doctors do for these children? They had been
born with not one defect, but four. Their lungs were starved of
blood because the valve leading from the right heart chamber
had narrowed and thickened. This caused the lower chamber
to balloon because the blood piled up. To complicate matters,
the septum dividing the chambers of both sides of the heart
had split, and through this blood shunted from the left ventricle
into the right. The aorta, carrying blood to all the arteries of
the body, had been misplaced and stole some of the blood from
the right side of the heart. Described first by the Marseilles
doctor, Fallot, in 1888, this quadruple series of inborn defects
presented the surgeon and the physician with an almost insuperable problem. Fallot dubbed the condition "La Maladie
Bleue" and his description of the four malformations earned
this heart condition the name of the Tetralogy of Fallot. With
its incidence of one case in 8,500 births, the Blue-Baby disease
had come to be one of the biggest single problems facing the
heart surgeon.

Without opening the heart, closing the hole, relieving the

stricture in the pulmonary valve and correcting the displaced main blood vessel, there seemed nothing doctors could do. So children who came into hospitals and clinics during their many crises passed a few weeks in an oxygen tent and then went home to wait for the next attack.

Many of these children came to the heart clinic at the Harriet Lane Home in Baltimore and were seen there by a physician called Helen B. Taussig. Several things struck Dr. Taussig as curious about these children. Their lungs, for example—they did not pick up oxygen in the way they should. This, she reasoned, could be due to the depletion of blood caused by the blocked valve in the right heart chamber. Increase the blood supply, the oxygen uptake would rise, health would improve and the livid look would disappear.

Dr. Taussig noticed something else. Some Blue Babies had been born not only with the classic quartet of defects, but with an open duct between the aorta and the pulmonary arteries—of the type on which Gross had first operated successfully. These children seemed to fare much better than others . . . until the duct was tied off, or sectioned and stitched.

The surgical closing of the duct in fact turned infants with some degree of breathlessness into Blue Babies; in not a few cases they died after this corrective operation. Obviously the blood shunted through this inborn defect, by-passing the right pumping chamber of the heart, did help by increasing the blood supply to the lungs. If this proved right, then could not an artificial duct be created by fusing a major artery to the blood vessels which served the lungs?

Dr. Taussig discussed her observations with Dr. Alfred Blalock, 45-year-old Professor of Surgery and Director of the Johns Hopkins surgery department. This gifted surgeon agreed with her that if they could detour blood from the main blood vessel to the lungs it would save many of these hopeless children.

Blalock happened to be one of the few men in the world with experience in creating artificial short-circuits between blood vessels. Six years before, at the Vanderbilt University, Nashville, Tennessee, he and another surgeon, Dr. Sanford Levy, had carried out experiments to divert blood from major arteries to one of the lungs. The surgeons wanted to see whether the lung could withstand blood coming from the left side of the heart at four times the pressure from the normal side. Not only did they find that the lung remained healthy; the circulation in the rest of the body did not suffer from the procedure.

With healthy animals they could create a short-circuit of blood from one part to another; with someone's child it became a more serious matter, bristling with snags. Could they assume that a major artery could be borrowed without setting up trouble in the part of the body it nourished? Would the heart and lungs, already weakened by defects, accept such radical surgery? Could they block off the blood supply to one of the lungs for half an hour or more without injuring it? Finally, the suturing of one artery to another faced the surgeon with an intricate piece of surgical *petit point*.

Blalock spent another year working on animals to prove that the human body would support the removal of various arteries. He went through the operating procedure, perfecting the technique and devising new methods of stitching one artery to another. He decided that one of the three major arteries branching from the aorta to the arms, neck and head could be used to construct the artificial by-pass, and several months after his experiments prepared to accept the first patient. The two collaborators had no problem in finding cases.

The first of their Blue Babies had been born in the obstetric wing of Blalock's own hospital, on the 3rd August, 1943, just a year before he thought himself ready to operate. She was a premature baby, weighing no more than two and a quarter

pounds at birth. The bluish tint of her lips and skin, the murmur over her heart disappeared in the first months and she was
discharged when four months old. But at eight months she
came back suffering from a heart attack following a meal.
The livid pallor had increased; so had the blowing heart sound.
To the doctors it became clear they were dealing with a
Tetralogy of Fallot. By that time the strain of eating caused the
child to roll up her eyes, turn blue and often faint. She was
described as poorly nourished and developed, her eyes had a
glassy look, her lips were blue and examination revealed an
enlarged heart. Three weeks in an oxygen tent brought a slight
improvement, but her case was considered hopeless and she
was sent home.

In the middle of October the girl came into hospital again.
During her six weeks in the ward her condition deteriorated,
she refused to touch food, and it became obvious that if
surgery had nothing to offer she would die.

Professor Blalock and Dr. Taussig had by now perfected
their technique. It had stood the scrutiny of rigorous tests,
and they decided to try to save the girl.

On the 29th of November, 1944, Blalock performed the
operation. He found the pulmonary artery normal, but one
of the veins bringing fresh blood from the lungs appeared to be
smaller than usual. Skilfully, he clamped off one of the lung
arteries and between his two pairs of forceps made an incision.
The artery nearest to the pulmonary vein was cut, tied off at its
top end. Blalock then brought the lower part down to join it
with the artery going to the lungs. The stitching took half an
hour, during which time the lung was out of circulation. When
the surgeon released the clamps he listened for the tell-tale thrill
from the heart which would prove that flow in the pulmonary
artery had been boosted with blood from the aorta. It came,
and he closed the chest.

But the troubles of the surgeon had by no means finished

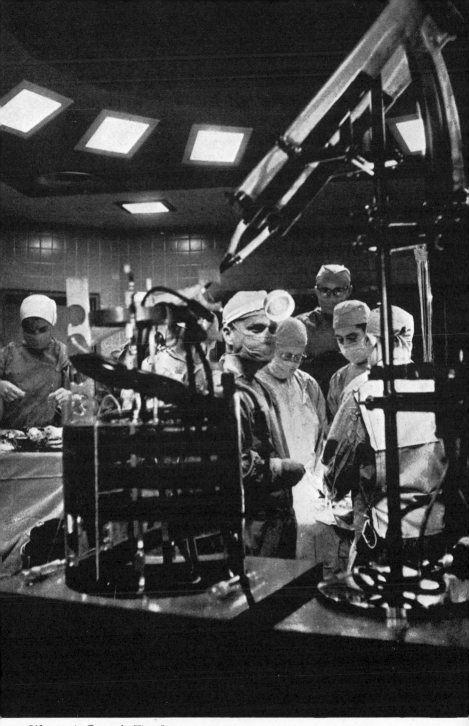

Dr. Lillehei, with head lamp, watches the blood flowing down the plastic column of his
machine to be oxygenated and passed through the helix and returned to the patient

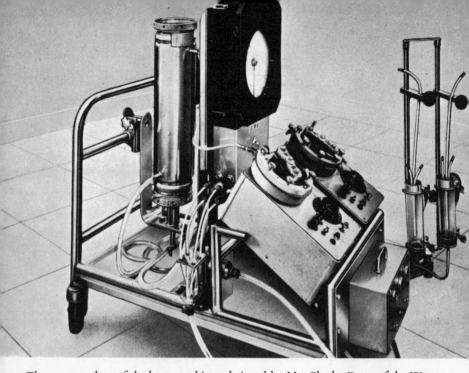

The most modern of the heart machines, designed by Mr. Charles Drew of the Westminster Hospital and the APV engineering firm. Consisting of twin pumps and a cooling
cylinder, the Drew machine can bring down the patient's blood from 98° F. to 50° F. in
half an hour

The forerunner of the modern heart-lung machines. This model was built by International Business Machines for Dr. John H. Gibbon. The machine was successful, though
early failures drove it back into the laboratory and workshop. Gibbon used two mechanical pumps, seen at the top of the apparatus, to replace the heart and his "lung" was
several sheets of wire mesh placed at the right side

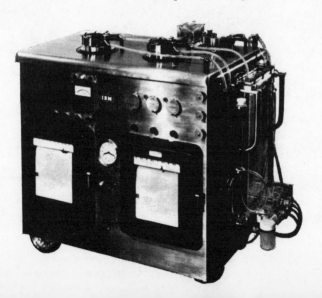

when he placed the last stitches. He and Dr. Taussig summed up the post-operative care of the girl in three words: "This was stormy." For two weeks, she lay between life and death; six doctors took it in turns to watch the child as she lay in the oxygen tent. The left arm in which the circulation had diminished became noticeably colder than the other, with no pulse at the wrist. But the lungs gave most trouble. With the extra burden on them they collapsed repeatedly and had to be re-expanded. But, two months after the operation, the baby had gained weight, her colour had improved, the heart and lungs were sound and the lack of circulation gave no cause for worry. On the 25th of January, 1945, she was discharged from hospital —the first successful Blue-Baby case.

Two other operations which followed the first confirmed their technique and allowed them to publish the results. The Blalock-Taussig report in the *Journal of the American Medical Association* will go down as a classic piece of co-operation between the physician and the surgeon, a model of clinical clarity and a piece of brilliant surgery. Their description of the medial detection, the surgical technique and their three cases, ran to more than 15,000 words. Blalock had textbook sketches made of his method of joining the end of one artery to the side of another so that almost any chest surgeon might attempt the operation after reading the paper. Blalock travelled widely, demonstrating the operation, and shortly after the war came to Britain with film of his technique which stimulated British surgeons to adopt the Blue-Baby technique. In the years before the machines arrived to make open-heart surgery a reality, the Blalock-Taussig operation gave relief to thousands of babies and acquitted many of an early death sentence.

Other surgeons noted the improvement in Blue Babies after the Blalock operation, quickly seized on his technique and began to practise and look for methods of improving it. Inevitably, one surgeon, Dr. Willis J. Potts of Chicago

University, devised just as ingenious a method of by-passing the blood from the main body channel into the lung artery.

These two arteries branch out of the heart together, the pulmonary artery passing beneath the arch of the main artery. They are connected at birth, before the patent duct closes, and therefore made the ideal choice for the surgeon who wanted to connect them again. The difficulty: cutting off the supply of these two arteries to link them would certainly kill the patient. To attempt to connect them without clamping would mean massive blood letting, and again death.

Potts gave a great deal of thought to the problem, and then arrived at the solution: pinch parts of the two arteries together to squeeze the blood out of them and then join them. All that he needed were the right instruments. These he devised—a pair of wide tongs which encircled the arteries. The end of the clamp he fashioned like an open vice to crimp off part of the artery in the way a seamstress might take in a tuck. In this way, Potts could ensure that blood flowed through the arteries and still leave himself a clamped portion on which to work. He used one pair of special forceps to pinch the lung artery, another to immobilize a section of the main artery. In the bloodless parts he made first a slit, then punched a round hole and brought the two incisions together. It demanded a button-stitching technique of very great skill, working on arteries which slipped and slid while the surgeon was hampered by rubber gloves and had to use needle forceps. It says much for surgeons that the operation became standard in hundreds of theatres.

Other variations of the Blalock and Potts operations exist. This "by-pass" technique, though never considered more than a makeshift treatment for Blue Babies, has saved the lives of thousands of children throughout the world. It certainly ranks with the greatest feats of surgery.

The grand illusion that the heart was a frail and delicate

structure was disappearing: the Second World War gave it the final push. From every front came stories of British, American and Russian surgeons, often working with primitive equipment, removing bullets and shrapnel from the heart and its surroundings and getting away with this life-and-death surgery.

Perhaps the strangest medical record belongs to Dr. Dwight Emary Harken, of Harvard Medical School, who was working in the South of England when the D-Day casualties began to arrive in their hundreds by boat and plane. In ten months, at the 160th General Hospital, Harken and his colleagues cut out 134 pieces of shrapnel from the heart and its blood vessels. His work, carried out at the height of the invasion and practically in "bomb alley", won Harken the Military Cross—and the distinction of proving that the heart was tough enough to be opened, manhandled and shut without rebelling. Harken ventured into the chambers of the heart thirteen times to grasp and remove shrapnel and splinters which would have killed soldiers. What might be called "The Case of the Wandering Missile" is a surgical classic in itself.

One of the first heart casualties to come into the field hospital from France was a 29-year-old infantry sergeant who had been wounded on the 21st of July at Saint-Lô. The burly sergeant was shipped back with a neat hole in his chest and a piece of shell somewhere behind the wound. The X-rays revealed that the oblong fragment, about three-quarters of an inch in size, was pulsing inside the right chamber of the heart. Heart tracings confirmed the presence of the missile. Though it lay in the middle of the ventricle and did not seem to interfere with the heart action it might have blocked the outflow or caused a fatal clot to form. So Harken decided he would attempt an operation to pluck it out of the chamber.

On the 15th of August he opened the sergeant's chest and exposed the heart, slitting the pericardium to reveal the right chamber. In this he made a small slit through which he pushed forceps, while with his free hand he guided these towards the shrapnel. Gripping the missile in the forceps he began to pull it gently through the hole.

But the heart muscle, still pounding and pumping blood into the lungs, wriggled against the forceps and snatched the piece of shell out of the surgeon's grasp. For some minutes he played hide and seek with the missile . . . then, unable to feel it he gave up and closed the chest.

However, another set of X-rays picked it up—lying this time in the top right chamber just above where the veins emptied blood into it.

For the second operation, on the 16th of November, Harken decided to approach the heart from the right side, and laid the sergeant on his left side. He opened the upper chamber, saw the jagged shrapnel, felt it . . . and watched it slip away once more. When they looked at the X-rays they found it had gone back into the lower chamber through the three-leaved valve.

For another three months they waited, and then tried a third operation on the 19th of February at the sergeant's request. One thing they noticed when they opened the heart; the previous wounds had healed solidly. The right chamber of the heart had, however, a flabby unhealthy look at its point. Judging that the muscle damage had been done by the foreign body Harken opened the heart and this time grasped the piece of metal and withdrew it carefully through the incision. Out it came, a small black body with saw-toothed edges.

The sergeant left hospital with nothing to show for his ordeal but a couple of operation scars. His heart appeared none the worse for having given houseroom to a piece of shrapnel for the best part of a year. Harken's was, without doubt, the most dramatic experience of the war with heart and chest wounds and he quelled any doubts that might have remained about the ability of the heart to shrug aside the most robust surgical treatment. Back at the Harvard Medical School, Harken became one of the first to tackle the recalcitrant mitral valve in earnest after the war and was only just behind Dr. Charles Bailey who did the first successful operation to clear the valve. But Harken's example, and the miraculous tales which came in from other battle fronts, paved the way for an all-out assault on the heart after the war.

6

The "Blind" Heart Surgeons

BRITISH interest in heart surgery, which had languished or trailed behind American work since Souttar's solitary gamble, came to life dramatically with the achievements of one surgeon. Russell Brock, a brilliant and courageous operator, chafed at the way in which surgeons everywhere left the heart alone while tackling the blood vessels round it.

A forthright man, Brock declared that his colleagues had failed to follow up Rehn's early success with sufficient determination. He complained of the indirect methods and said that few operations had been done on the substance of the heart— save for the removal of foreign bodies. Where the valves had closed it should not be impossible to devise techniques to relieve them; surgery was wanting if it could not clear simple mechanical obstructions.

The developments in surgery, anaesthesia, blood transfusion and oxygen treatment had enhanced the prospects of success in heart surgery. "The time has now come to try the matter again," said Brock in the *British Medical Journal*. Following his own injunction, the surgeon evolved a daring and ingenious solution to the problem of entering the main pumping compartment of the heart, and pulled off a series of dazzling operations which altered the character of heart surgery for a decade.

Brock knew and had practised Blalock's famous Blue-Baby operation. He paid great tribute to the surgeon and physician who had created and brought it to such a pitch of surgical excellence. But was it the real answer for these crippled children? No; at best it gave patients a longer expectancy of life. On the other hand it left an open duct which, if found as an inborn defect, was invariably closed. There arose, too, the risk that a child might outgrow the borrowed artery from which its lungs drew their blood and a further operation would have to follow.

Brock, working at Guy's Hospital with Dr. Maurice Campbell, one of the country's most talented cardiologists, reasoned that he could improve on Blalock's indirect method by a frontal attack on the valve which caused most of the trouble. Several people argued that stretching the fused lung-artery valve might leave those children who had the dreaded quartet of heart defects worse off than before; others maintained the direct approach would not relieve deep-seated stenosis.

At Guy's they went ahead. The surgeon called in an instrument expert and had him develop a new cardioscope with which he could examine the valve while it opened and shut within the heart. After three attempts with the new research tool, Brock reluctantly abandoned it, deciding that he and Campbell could assess the type of heart disease before and during the operation. From his observations he deduced that as the three petals of the pulmonary valve close, they are often pushed into the pulmonary artery like the point of a pencil. He foresaw no difficulty in dividing the cusps to allow the valve to vent more blood into the lungs. Brock refused to rely on the finger technique used by Souttar and the Americans who took up his mitral valve technique. A London manufacturing company listened to his ideas and came back with two instruments which would divide the valve without too much blood-letting from the main heart chambers.

His valvulotome had a thin stem, flattening at the end into a spear-shaped blade with two cutting edges. A tear-drop point acted as a probe. Those and a set of forceps with fine, curved blades made up his special instruments.

Only one question confronted the surgeon. Could he achieve what no one else had: open a main chamber of the heart and get away with it? Three cases waited for him to operate, among them an 11-year-old girl called Gwenda.

The youngest of eight children, Gwenda had typical Blue Baby symptoms. Before she was six months old her parents had noted her blue lips. Soon after her first birthday she began walking, but her parents saw that she would take a few paces and then squat to regain her energy. More than 100 yards tired her; half a mile left her exhausted. When they brought her to Guy's her blue tint had become obvious, and her fingers showed the clubbing typical of many of these children.

The surgeon described Gwenda's heart as sabot-shaped. From it came a loud murmur in the region of the pulmonary valve. The right heart chamber was enlarged. The surgeon and physician diagnosed Fallot's Tetralogy—the condition which many doctors contended could not be helped by opening the lung valve.

Brock decided to operate on the 19th of February, 1948. He approached the heart through the left side of the chest. Reckoning that the operation might succeed with his new technique, he placed two rows of stitches in the wall of the right heart chamber. An assistant held these tight while the surgeon cut through the thick heart muscle. As he passed the valvulotome he felt the pressure of the fused valves against the instrument before he carried it through into the lung artery. The stretching forceps were then inserted and opened wide.

The method worked. Only the condition of the patient worried Brock and his colleagues. Gwenda still had poor colour; her pulse had weakened and then improved; her blood pressure had fallen slightly during the operation. It took a whole week of careful nursing in an oxygen tent after the operation to bring colour back into her face. But a few days later the girl got out of bed and visited the adjoining ward. They were having a birthday party in the children's ward at

Guy's the day that Gwenda got up. Gone were the blue lips and the pale face; a pink-cheeked little girl enjoyed herself with the other children.

Three months later, the surgeon saw the child with her mother, who reported that Gwenda could now run, something she had never done before the operation. Her nails were now pink where before they had been blue. The surgeon in the terse footnote to his report of the operation remarked: "The result of valvulotomy has been most encouraging." In five weeks he performed three similar operations to confirm his success.

Brock had more than made surgical history; he gave British heart surgeons a lead they had long lacked and encouraged even the Americans to dare instead of hesitating.

The British surgeon devised a whole range of special instruments for "blind" heart surgery. To stretch and split fused valve cups, he designed a set of right-angled forceps with scissor handles whose bullet-shaped point opened out like flower petals. Pushing the point of the instrument into the valve and extending the steel flanges severed the joined edges of blocked valves.

Where the narrow mouth of the valve had furred up like a corroded pipe, Brock used a special punch. The blunt end of this punch could be thrust forward to unsheath sharp blades which gripped the excess tissue lining the valve entrance. As the punch closed it nipped out the tissue, relieving the blockage. For mitral valve work, the British surgeon designed a finger scalpel. Fitted to a ring which could be slipped over the forefinger, the knife could then be used as the surgeon felt any defects in the valve.

Brock's surgical feats have saved thousands of patients from distress or death through heart defects. For these he received a knighthood in 1954. The next year, talking to leading heart surgeons from all over the world at Detroit, he recalled the dark days when he had four successive deaths among women patients while they were developing their heart surgery techniques.

"Despair stalked before us and everyone's morale was low," said the British surgeon. "I remember saying to my team that we could do only one of two things—give up or go on—that it was impossible to give up as we were certainly in the right. The only thing, therefore, that we should do was to go on. We did continue and had thirty consecutive successful cases."

Though he published his results before anyone else, Brock found he had not got there first. Less than two miles away, in the Middlesex Hospital, one of his contemporaries had conceived exactly the same idea for pulmonary valvulotomy two months before. T. Holmes Sellors, a gifted and distinguished surgeon and a year older than Brock, wrote his report of the operation before his colleague's appeared; but it went into print in the *Lancet* a fortnight afterwards.

Neither surgeon knew about the other's technique, though their methods were almost identical. The patient, a youth of 20, came to Sellors with tuberculosis and the blue tint and drumstick fingers indicating a bad heart. The surgeon knew that the TB would not clear until he had done something about the heart condition. They diagnosed the four Fallot defects, and decided that the Blalock by-pass operation might help.

On the 14th of December, 1947, when the chest was opened, the surgeon saw that the lung and main arteries were joined by an open duct. Pinching this closed with his fingers did nothing to quieten the thrill over the heart, so they decided to try to prise apart the blocked pulmonary valve. Sellors chose to enter the heart at the base of this valve with a long knife used for cutting tendons. He placed holding stitches round the point of entry and then forced the knife through until it found the stuck valve. Guiding it with the left hand he managed to sever the fused leaflets of the valve. Immediately, the thrill caused by the blockage abated. There was little blood loss, the patient recovered and was discharged to be treated for his tuberculosis.

With these successes, heart surgery suddenly seemed to

burgeon into an art in itself. The difficult pulmonary valve had fallen to the knife; but still the mitral valve on which Souttar had made his sole attempt about a quarter of a century before remained obstinate. However, only a month after Brock and Sellors announced their results, the Americans finally triumphed over mitral stenosis.

It was on the 10th of June that Dr. Charles P. Bailey reported that he had split the two valves which blocked the inflow into the main chamber of the heart. He had tried before—twice. Each time something had happened to frustrate him, though, like Souttar and others, he knew that the surgery presented no insuperable problem.

To carry out the operation on a 24-year-old woman, Bailey designed a small, curved knife which looked like a crochet pin with keen edges. He practised using this between the fingers of his hand which he encased in two pairs of rubber gloves. He adopted Souttar's technique of opening the flap of the right atrium, pulling it over his fingers like a glove and then drawing the sharp, hooked end of his knife along the fused line of the valve leaves.

His success was dramatic. The woman, who had severe disease of the valve, went home from the Episcopal Hospital in Philadelphia almost completely cured. Bailey, Professor of Surgery at the Hahnemann Medical College, began doing mitral surgery as a routine. Quickly following his lead came Dwight Harken at Harvard, and a couple of months later, Brock in London was splitting the leaves of mitral valves either with his finger or a fingered knife.

The roadblocks which had kept surgeons out of the heart for centuries had finally been broken down. The success of the pioneers with valve operations encouraged surgeons every-where to venture into the heart. And in the decade after these first cases the long queues of people with valvular disease shrank as the operation became commonplace.

But there were still advances in the technique, this time from Edinburgh University where a surgeon and a doctor devised a bolder and more effective road into the heart valves.

The finger technique had worked wonders. But, even when a knife was used to cut the valves along their fused edges, the approach through the upper chamber of the heart proved tricky. The finger often did not complete the job of tearing the valve leaves apart; the knife often cut them in the wrong place. The business of levering open a stubborn and stenosed valve sometimes did incidental damage to the heart, and occasionally stopped it beating. Using the type of dilator which could be placed in the valve and then expanded involved the risk of tangling it in the "heart strings" holding the mitral valve firm.

The two Edinburgh men, Andrew Logan, a surgeon, and Richard Turner, the physician, turned their attention to the alternative route—through the left ventricle. This, the thickest, strongest of the heart's four chambers, had been punctured before, but only accidentally or with great trepidation. Analogous to removing a tap before shutting off the water main, the ventricular puncture did not suggest itself to most surgeons as a likely method of mitral valve surgery.

The Edinburgh University pair decided they would do a "pincer operation"—slit the ventricle at the lower pointed end of the heart; at the same time they would pierce the left, upper chamber. Through the ventricle they would thrust a knife and, with a finger inserted in the atrial hole, they could guide the blade along the stuck valve cusps. It sounded perfect —until they came to practise it. Doubts began to hit both men and for a year from the 17th of June, 1954—the first time they tried the route through the lower chamber—they used it only sporadically.

But gradually they saw that their method had distinct advantages over the others. They also acquired a dilating instrument designed by a London surgeon, Oswald S. Tubbs, who did the first patent ductus operation in Britain. This instrument stretched the valve much further than others they had used—and the results started to improve. Such an operation called for skill and courage in the early days. But in five years, the two Edinburgh doctors performed 438 operations through the auricle and ventricle and found their patients felt better, though the mortality was slightly higher. Other surgeons, in Glasgow, took up the method and had fewer deaths than with the finger-and-knife technique.

To carry out the Logan-Turner operation the surgeon works with both hands. When he exposes the heart, he clamps off the left, upper chamber to prevent blood loss, nicks it just enough to insert a gloved finger. With this, he "reads" the valve and then knows what setting to apply to the dilator. The left hand he uses to stab through the ventricle and to insert the long dilator. He guides the point into the small orifice of the valve, then slowly opens it by pressing on the ends which have the shape of pliers. Blood loss from the ventricle is controlled merely by pressing on the slit with the thumb.

With their triumphs over the valvular defects surgeons could now cope with the infective heart diseases. Mitral valve disease, which gives most trouble, remains a problem since many thousands of children suffer yearly from rheumatic fever, and it has been reckoned by health authorities that one out of every two cases have a legacy of heart disease. Men who operated on long-term and advanced cases of valve disease were often amazed at how the heart would suddenly take out a new lease of life, and how quickly it recovered from man-handling in the operating theatre.

Valvular disease might have fallen to the surgeon—but he still had to tackle the dozen different types of inborn disease. In the years which followed the first valve operations the heart would suffer quite a few knocks and shocks—and still show that it was the most powerful muscle in the body.

7

The First Robot

IN A matter of nine years surgeons had built up an impressive
record of successful heart operations. The Gross technique
had become routine, so had the Blalock-Taussig technique
of funnelling blood through a by-pass into the lungs. Charles
Bailey and Russell C. Brock were doing dozens of operations
on the mitral and the pulmonary valves, saving and prolonging
lives.

But the majority of these methods lacked two things: a
direct look at the inside of the heart and the assurance that
the organ would not falter and fail while the surgeon worked
on it.

The operations for open duct defects and to correct Blue-
Baby conditions did not involve the main chambers of the
heart. But with difficult mitral and pulmonary valves, the
surgeons literally had to grope until they became skilled
enough to find and repair the defects blindfold.

While surgeons perfected valve operations, the cardiologists
were charting the more serious malformations inside the heart.
Out of all the children with heart disease about one in fifty
was a victim of some inborn defect which crippled the mechanism of the organ. Statisticians estimated that six children out
of every 1,000 born had some congenital heart defect; taking
the still births, the figure rose to eight in a thousand. These
were killing deformities, and thirty-two out of every hundred
children did not live beyond a month. Another nine out of this
hundred died before their first birthday. Those who did survive

lived pathetic existences and all too often died before they were thirty years of age.

These congenital diseases occurred while the heart was developing in the embryo. From a simple tube-like structure the heart transforms itself into the four-chambered pump between the fifth and eighth weeks of pregnancy—and it is then that the defects appear. How and why? Most suspicion rests on the infectious illnesses which mothers suffer during these vital weeks. Of these diseases, german measles, one of the mildest, is thought to be the biggest culprit. This clue to heart malformations follows research done by an Australian eye specialist in 1941.

The specialist, Dr. N. M. Gregg, found in the spring of this year that his clinic was filling with an unusually large number of children showing a form of eye trouble he had hardly ever seen. These "blind spots" in the eyes appeared at birth and Dr. Gregg therefore concluded that something might have happened during pregnancy. Though interested mainly in the eye trouble, Gregg noticed that some of the babies were deaf; others seemed slow in speaking and in their general development. And, most surprising of all, among them appeared a high proportion of children with typical Blue-Baby symptoms. Gregg made inquiries among the parents and discovered that in almost every case the mothers of these children had caught german measles in the first, second or third month of pregnancy. Could this benign illness have attacked the foetus and caused the inborn defects? Gregg thought so, and made a report to this effect. At first, American and British doctors were inclined to dismiss the notion, but later research confirmed Gregg's deductions. The whole story of congenital defects still has to be unravelled, but german measles forms a big part of it.

The most common of these deformities is the hole in the heart between the two ventricles. More than one in five crippled children have this condition where the thick septum dividing the right and left ventricle has not formed properly. In rare cases, the child has no division at all between the two pumping chambers. A patent duct comes next on the list of congenital malformations, then the Blue Babies and a list of other conditions, including holes between the upper heart chambers and constriction of the aorta.

The valve conditions would yield to "blind surgery". But who would attempt to repair a hole even between the upper chambers of the heart while it was still pumping? To attempt surgery on these conditions meant opening the organ, something which made even the most intrepid men shudder. But some of them began asking: could we not cut the heart out of the circulation long enough to make open-heart surgery possible? Two ideas had already been mooted; the heart-lung machine and hypothermia. This latter method of cooling the body had been tried experimentally and did extend the time that the heart might be made amenable to surgery on its chambers. The machine which would take over from the heart and lungs was still a dream.

Both ideas certainly bristled with problems. Hypothermia seemed on the face of things simpler than making a mechanical heart and lungs. Hibernating animals showed that they could shut off the consciousness for months, lower their temperatures, eat and drink nothing—and awake after this Rip van Winkle treatment none the worse. The human body slows down during sleep. If it were cooled down twenty degrees or so, then the brain and other vital organs would not starve or die for lack of oxygen. Several experimental operations had shown hypothermia to be feasible. But it was the machines which made the first impact on surgery.

Before the war most medical men would have dismissed the heart lung machine as a piece of science fiction. Some doctors toyed with the suggestion and then decided that it lay beyond medicine and engineering.

The idea of making a pump do the work of the heart had, in fact, been mooted as far back as 1812 by a doctor who thought it would save people with failing hearts. As a brainwave, it sounded simple; but the doctors who began drafting plans for such a pump soon saw that between its conception and execution lay a maze of problems. Only one of them persisted through the inter-war years with his ideas of creating such a device.

Dr. John H. Gibbon met the usual rebuffs and disappointments when he proposed building a pump which would duplicate the heart action, and a pair of mechanical lungs to keep the blood charged with life-giving oxygen. Three years before Gross tied off the patent ductus, Gibbon had advocated such a machine to make open-heart surgery a reality. In 1937, two years later, he had planned the machine and merely waited for funds and backing to build it. Gibbon found few supporters, and for years preached to stony-faced colleagues who listened without credulity and did nothing.

The young Philadelphia surgeon had nothing much to guide him. Two Russian medical scientists had considered the problems of isolating the heart and had, in 1926, designed a crude machine to carry out experiments on animals. The scientists, Professor S. Brukhonenko and S. Tchetchuline, succeeded during the next two years in keeping animals alive with this machine, but then discontinued their work. Gibbon, too, might have given up; it took him nearly twenty years to convince the medical profession that he could build a heart and lungs out of steel and glass. For most of this time he was planning and discussing the problem himself.

Gibbon first saw his heart-lung machine as a "prop" to tide patients over emergencies. The heart might flag when its valves failed to do their work; its main muscle might tire if starved of blood; or the lungs might choke. In all these situations the patient might be plugged temporarily into a machine which would keep feeding blood and oxygen into the body while the crisis lasted.

As he said in the early days, "The other reason for building and perfecting such a machine is the hope that some day it might take over the entire work of the heart and lungs for a period of time long enough to permit a surgeon to open the chambers of the heart and to perform operations inside it. Under those conditions it might be possible to correct malformations which sometimes are present at birth, or to graft in new tissue to take the place of damaged valves, which often occur as a result of rheumatic fever.

"At present it is impossible to open the heart and perform these operations under direct vision, because the heart is full of blood and must keep the blood circulating through the body. By-passing the blood around the heart and lungs would allow the surgeon to open the heart without losing blood and to operate in the empty inside chambers, knowing that the job of the heart and lungs was being temporarily performed by a machine."

Mechanically the heart machine presented few problems. As a pump, the heart keeps about twelve pints of blood coursing through the body to the myriad cells. Substitute two pumps working in phase, one to drive blood through the lungs, the other to push it out through the arteries, and you can replace the heart, Gibbon said. Here, he gave a warning about blood. The heart, however hard it squeezes, does not damage the sensitive blood cells; the pump, likewise, must not injure the cells which pick up and transfer the oxygen which body cells breathe. Nor should it allow the blood to clot and stick to the machine. So the heart pumps must treat the blood with care, their parts should not clog with blood and should be easy to maintain and sterilize.

The two pumps would operate thus: one would suck blood out of the great veins which pour it into the heart and from there to the lungs; the other would inject the fresh blood from the machine into a major artery as the heart does.

But how does man create a stand-in for the lungs? Like giant sea-sponges the lungs, through their countless millions of microscopic air sacs, revitalize the blood in the body by filtering the oxygen out of the air we breathe, at the same time giving up the waste carbon dioxide gas from the cells. Their walls, many times thinner than tissue-paper, would spread out flat to cover the whole of an operating-room floor. The surgeon and engineer who wanted to charge blood with oxygen as it flowed through the heart pump would have to bring it into contact with a surface as wide if not wider than the lungs.

Gibbon wrestled with this problem and concluded that if the blood flow through the pump were passed over flat surfaces and saturated with pure oxygen this would revitalize it. Five systems of pump he tried before settling for a large, bright metal box on wheels, five-and-a-half feet long and four feet high, designed to the surgeon's specifications and presented to him by the International Business Machine Corporation.

The "heart" of the machine consisted of two roller pumps which squeezed blood through plastic tubes in the way that a mangle wrings water out of clothes.

The "lung" through which the blood passed stood at the end of the cabinet in a long plastic box. Its six wafers of stainless-steel mesh spread the blood over their surface while oxygen was blown over them. In front of the box four automatic recording charts told the operating team how much oxygen and carbon dioxide the blood contained, the volume of blood passing through the machine, its temperature and pressure.

No less important was the method which Gibbon devised for cutting the heart out of the circulation while the machine assumed its functions. He made stainless-steel cannulae, small hollow tubes, to fit the blood vessels entering and leaving the heart. He devised a method for emptying the heart of spent blood from its own coronary arteries, and for preventing an airlock in the arteries. In 1952 the machine was ready for its trials—on animals.

By the spring of 1953, Gibbon and his collaborators were presenting the results of repairing defects inside the hearts of animals while their circulation had been sustained by his machine. Slowly and methodically the team at the Jefferson Medical College, Philadelphia, toiled over the techniques of tying off the heart, opening up the atria and the ventricles and stitching and patching defects. Their work convinced them that they could move the machine into the operating theatre and take the heart cases which were considered beyond "blind" surgery.

In March, 1953, came the first case—a baby of 15 months weighing only 11 lbs. who had severe congestive heart failure. According to the physicians and surgeons his trouble arose from a hole in his heart between the two upper chambers. This, they said, would cause a blood shunt from the left into the right atrium and reduce the volume of blood to the arteries.

The surgeons carried out the drill they had evolved with animals. The small heart of the child was bared, the terminals of the machine were plugged into the main veins and a major artery. The right side of the heart was then opened up and the surgeons began to probe for the gap between the atria. They found none. They could do nothing but close the heart. The child died soon after the operation.

Was the machine at fault? No, it behaved perfectly; but the surgeons and doctors had missed a large open duct of the type which they could easily have repaired without its aid.

Two months later, on May 6th, they tried again, this time with an older patient, a girl of 18. Until six months before the operation she had been a normal, healthy girl. Suddenly, the signs of a heart defect appeared which brought her into hospital three times and put her life in peril.

Gibbon and his team decided to attempt surgery with the machine. But before the operation they explored the heart by passing a catheter through the girl's arm vein into the right upper chamber. The samples of mixed fresh and spent blood proved they were dealing this time with a large hole between the two upper chambers through which fresh blood was ebbing at the rate of seventeen pints a minute. This endangered the left side of the heart and would have meant heart failure had the gap been left open.

The surgeons opened the right upper chamber of the heart and slipped two metal plugs into the veins, draining the top and bottom of the body. They inserted another cannula into one of the arteries leading from the top of the heart. Then they switched the girl's body on to the machine.

For twenty-six minutes the pumps kept her alive while her heart was isolated from the circulation. During that time the right upper chamber of the heart was incised and there, between the two auricles, they found what they had suspected— a gaping hole through which blood had escaped. Quickly they stitched it with silk thread and then closed the heart and chest.

Two months later, the girl came back. The heavy "blup" sound of the murmur had disappeared, her colour had returned to its healthy pink. And the tube, slipped up her vein into the heart, revealed that the blood shunt had gone.

It seemed that Gibbon had proved his machine, that now heart surgeons could venture with impunity into the interior of the organ and make hole-in-the-heart surgery safe.

But the next two cases made Gibbon and his colleagues think again. They were both girls of 18 months, and they came into the operating theatre shortly after the successful case had been re-examined. Both died following their operations, but in neither case could death be attributed to the machine. One child had heart failure before the heart-lung machine began to work; the other had such gross heart malformations that the surgeons could attempt nothing.

These set-backs, however, drove the Gibbon apparatus out of the operating theatre and back into the laboratory. The failures had also set the medical world wondering whether the patient could ever stand up to the shock of having his blood circulation kept going with a heart-lung machine, the opening of the heart and the running repairs to the organ itself.

Reluctantly, Gibbon had to retrace his steps over eighteen years of research and ponder what he might do to make the machine and the technique which went with it much safer for patients.

Now, of course, the surgeons know that the Gibbon machine suffered from no design flaws. The reason for its early failures lay more with the poor-risk patients, the failures in diagnosis and the lack of surgical team-work and technique which have to be built up round the machine. Two and a half years later, Gibbon's machine was performing faultlessly at the Mayo clinic in the hands of Dr. John W. Kirklin and his colleagues. But by then, other surgeons had broken into the field of heart-lung machines. And when a disappointed Gibbon was wondering where he went wrong, two of these surgeons had reached the point of trying their robots out on patients.

But Gibbon had achieved his object. Through his many published papers, his lectures and talks to fellow-surgeons, the principle of using machines to stand in for the heart and lungs found acceptance. A generous, unassuming man in a profession where many are uncharitable and jealous about their success, a humane man with a fine sense of humour, Gibbon deserves the name which his own profession bestowed on him: Father of the Heart-Lung Machine.

8

A Lesson from Poisoned Arrows

THE HEART surgeon could never have contemplated major operations on the open heart without the help of his specialist colleagues, the cardiologist and the anaesthetist, without the great advances which medical science had made in drugs, diagnostic and measuring instruments. Equally, the heart-lung machine could never have succeeded but for these gains.

Souttar, in 1925, paid tribute to his anaesthetist, John Challis, who took a risk with ether and chloroform, the original anaesthetics which had come into use in the middle of the nineteenth century. Until the late thirties of this century, anaesthetics stayed a rag-and-bottle science which took a back seat to the more glamorous surgery. But then, with the discovery of the barbiturates which could be injected into a vein, the "gas men" began to play a more prominent part in surgery.

We still do not understand how substances like ether, chloroform, morphine and the barbiturates act; but we now know a great deal about their effect on patients. When the surgeon considered his major onslaught on the heart with the aid of the machine, the anaesthetist could choose from a whole battery of drugs those which would ease the pain and the process of surgery. The science of keeping people asleep leaves little room for the accidents, which, unfortunately, could not be counted rare in earlier days.

A major heart operation when the machines were new was no light thing—both for surgeon and patient. So when the patient was "prepped", the anaesthetist gave him a shot of a morphine or barbiturate drug to quieten his apprehension and perhaps lessen the risk that the heart might rebel at surgery.

But the barbiturates needed long experience and delicate handling, so ether with several derivatives still remained the stock-in-trade of the anaesthetist. Much of the trouble with the original anaesthetics arose when the surgeon wanted complete relaxation in a patient, which meant giving him too much gas. Between deep anaesthesia and death often lay a fine line which was all too often crossed, and another "death through anaesthesia" was written into the statistics. Before the modern armoury of anaesthetics were developed, perhaps the biggest single advance came from a shy genius, Professor Arthur E. Guedel, of Wisconsin University. He laid down clinical standards for gauging the depth of unconsciousness and thus prevented many unnecessary deaths. He divided the depth of unconsciousness into seven planes, which are dunned into every modern medical student.

The big step for these merchants of oblivion came when they devised three-way anaesthesia—to keep the patient asleep; to kill his pain; and to relax the muscles for his sake and the surgeon's. Normally, the initial anaesthesia is induced with a barbiturate which is pushed into a vein. Then the anaesthetist switches over to his gas machine to feed through a breathing tube just enough nitrous oxide (laughing gas) and other agents to keep the patient under. While the patient sleeps the anaesthetist virtually paralyses most of his muscles with a drug called curare. Since his lungs, too, are defunct, the anaesthetist must take over the patient's breathing, which he does by squeezing air into the lungs from a rubber bladder.

Curare did not appear in the drug lists until after the war, but its history dates from antiquity and makes one of the fascinating tales of medicine. After his ill-fated quest of Eldorado, Sir Walter Raleigh brought back, with the potato and tobacco, some deadly poison with which, he said, South American Indians used to tip their arrows. For centuries explorers added to the news of how this poison killed quickly and dramatically. Alexander von Humboldt, the man who discovered the Humboldt Current, saw the hostile Amazon Indians prepare the poison from plants and wrote about it in 1807. A few years later, British traveller Charles Waterton went to South America in search of the "deadly wourali poison". Back he came with a quantity which he tried out on various animals.

The effect was extraordinary. The animals appeared to have slumbered quietly to death. Waterton was struck by one thing: the poison seemed to take all tension out of the muscles. He therefore turned to the problem of finding an antidote. It was a donkey which proved that the poison did not kill at all, but merely paralysed most of the body's muscles including the lungs. He deduced that the poison alone did not kill—only the respiratory failure. Waterton gave the animal a dose of curare and watched it apparently die in ten minutes. Then he made a slit in its windpipe, took a pair of household bellows, and began inflating the lungs. In two hours the ass had recovered. As a reward, it was billeted and fed for twenty-five years, until it died. Waterton called it Wouralia, after his name for the poison.

Curare lay on the shelf for fourteen years, until American psychiatrist A. E. Bennett ran it to earth in the medical literature and found a use for it. Patients whom the Nebraska doctor was treating with electric shock therapy for mental illness developed muscle spasm, and Bennett found that minute doses of the Indian poison relaxed their muscles.

Three years later, in Montreal, an anaesthetist, Dr. Harold Griffin, followed up Bennett's work and tried out the drug on animals with a view to introducing it into surgery. He discovered that the poison blocked the pathway from the nerves to the voluntary muscles and paralysed them until its effects wore off. Griffin also published the case history of a patient on whom he had tried the muscle relaxant successfully.

Another problem which the designer of heart-lung machines had to beat was blood clotting. As anyone knows who cuts a finger, blood will seal the cut in about seven minutes, form a clot and then a crust. So it would have happened to blood in the machines, with fatal outcome for the patient, had it not been for a substance discovered in the First World War by a medical student.

Heparin, so-called because it was isolated first from the liver, prolongs the clotting time by interfering with the chemical agents which cause the blood to congeal. Now obtained either from the liver or lungs, heparin is added to the blood used in machines to keep it flowing smoothly. A substance called pro-tamine neutralizes the action of heparin if there is danger of bleeding after operations.

As Brock had pointed out when he did the first pulmonary valve operations, the antibiotics had made surgery safer. When doctors considered taking the heart apart and repairing it, they had a whole range of penicillins and several other types of antibiotic to take care of the complications which might arise during and after the operations. The patient could be protected by a penicillin "umbrella" which ruled out the risk of infection during and after surgery.

With the advances in anaesthetics and other drugs came the fruition of heart exploration technique which Forssmann had discovered so long ago. Only a few years after the German doctor had used himself as a guinea pig, two American research workers took up the challenge of mapping the heart by remote control. Beginning with the principle that if they could sample blood from the right chambers of the heart they would know how efficiently it was working, the two doctors, André Cournand and Dickinson W. Richards, began to measure the content of oxygen and carbon dioxide in the breath of patients.

An accurate analysis of this would give them an index of the heart activity. But they abandoned this method, after three years of study, and turned to the tube-in-the-heart techniques.

At the Bellevue Hospital, New York, they soon translated Forssmann's life-and-death method into commonplace routine. A fine plastic tube could lie in the heart, they discovered, for more than twenty-four hours without discomforting the patient or producing infection or heart damage. From this tube they could draw samples of the blood which, when they had broken down the gases in them, gave the composition of the blood before the heart pushed it through the lungs. Comparing this with arterial blood they could tell if the heart was working efficiently.

During the war, Cournand and Richards were "called up" to study the effects of shock and blood loss, burns and injuries on service men sent to Bellevue Hospital. Their catheter technique showed how the heart could fail when a man had lost four or five of his ten pints of blood; how whole blood should be preferred to the plasma fraction for transfusions; how these transfusions might be piped directly into the heart through the plastic tube.

In the hands of Cournand and Richards, the catheter had become one of the most important diagnostic tools in cardiac surgery. Seizing on their lead, cardiologists began to probe not only the upper chamber of the right heart, but the lower chamber. A catheter, threaded through an arm or leg vein, might be pushed into the upper chamber, down past the three-leaved valve which stood at the opening to the right ventricle. Some experts became so clever with the tipped plastic tube they could have threaded a needle at long range with it. Their skill enabled them to sound the right heart to see if a pressure build-up indicated that the pulmonary valve had blocked; some even bent the catheter back on itself and probed through the valve into the main outflow artery to the lungs.

These catheter soundings told the surgeon much. If samples from the upper chambers showed mixed fresh and spent blood he could deduce a tear in the dividing wall between the atria. If the blood were mixed in the lower chambers then he faced repair of a ventricular defect in the septum or dividing wall. If the pressure in the main chamber of the right heart was high, he suspected a blocked outlet valve and perhaps a tear in the wall. From pressure and gas measurements the state of the heart could be fathomed.

The left side of the heart gave the cardiologist much more worry than the others. Only when he found a hole in the heart did he manage to push the plastic probe through into the left atrium or ventricle, and perhaps as far as the aortic valve. Another alternative was to slip the tube into an artery and push it past the aortic valve into the main left chamber and through the mitral valve into the left atrium.

The methods of sounding the left heart did not appeal to many surgeons. To slip a catheter through an artery against the blood flow was a risky procedure and might cause clotting of an artery, or damage to the aortic valve. To puncture the heart with a needle in the cause of diagnosis hardly seemed justifiable. At least, so it appeared to cardiologists at the National Heart Institute in Bethesda, Maryland. Dr. John Ross and two collaborators searched round for a less hazardous form of probing the left heart. Their final answer was a marvel in ingenuity. Determined to approach through a vein, Ross asked two firms to make a three-in-one catheter which could pierce the thick atrial wall of the heart without damaging it.

The catheter had three tubes. The outer was made of stiff nylon which in itself acted as the probe for the right heart. Threaded through this was a long, thin needle, curved at the end to ease its passage through the heart wall. The bore of this needle enveloped still another thread-like tube which would take samples and pressures of the left heart.

Ross made sure that his needle-in-the-heart method would leave no damage before he tried it on cardiac cases. The tube is slipped into the vein rising from the leg to join the main inflow into the right heart. When it has reached the right upper chamber and taken readings, the needle is pushed forward and gently thrust through into the left upper chamber. By paying out the third tube and skilfully manipulating it, this can be edged through the mitral valve into the main chamber of the heart. So, with one manœuvre, Ross managed to make a complete survey of the state of the heart. Before he published his results he made successful soundings of 150 patients with this catheter.

From its beginnings as an instrument which doctors shunned, the heart catheter has become a routine tool in any hospital which practises cardiac surgery. A patient runs no more risk with the tube-in-the-heart procedure than, say, giving a pint of blood. At several British hospitals, catheterization is carried out by laying the patient in front of an X-ray screen. He gets nothing in the way of anaesthetics; but to keep his mind off things he listens to music over special headphones while the staff run a tube into his heart, watch its progress on a T.V. screen, and draw off a few drops of blood. Even Forssmann must have smiled when he saw how the experiment which was maligned and derided had given birth to a whole new branch of diagnosis.

Various techniques run hand in hand with catheterization to elucidate heart disease. Substances such as iodine solutions which reflect X-rays can be injected into the blood stream and photographed as they pass through the chambers of the heart, thus giving indications of faults in valves or holes in the walls. Now, the doctor can study pictures of the heart while it moves by coupling X-rays to television equipment. These "live" views of the heart show how it will react to exertion, or even how it behaves during sleep.

To trace blood-flow through the heart and into its own net-work of arteries and veins, small amounts of short-lived radio-active materials can be infiltrated into the blood stream. Fol-lowed by sensitive Geiger counters, these substances will trace a pattern of blood flow which will tell whether the heart arteries are functioning normally.

The new diagnostic methods are backed by one of the oldest guides to the cardiologist—the electrocardiograph. The Dutch physician. Willem Einthoven, invented the first ECG appara-tus in 1903, using a string galvanometer to measure the tiny currents across heart muscle. These impulses make traces which are read like a form of shorthand by the cardiologist—but even he will admit the information is often confused or scanty about heart condition. The great British physiologist, Sir Thomas Lewis, identified certain of the ECG waves with electrical and muscular activity in the heart; but pioneer that he was, Lewis diagnosed his own coronary as indigestion in 1926. The ECG forms a vital part of the heart-surgeon's tools, telling him what he can expect to find when the operation is performed.

Another, equally useful machine is the electro-encephalo-graph, which records brain waves. Again, the EEG provokes much strife among specialists who read different meanings into the several types of currents which emanate from the brain. But hypothermia has elevated the EEG machine to an impor-tant role in surgery, for it tells when the oxygen supply to the vital brain cells is failing. In deep hypothermia it indicates when the cooling process has silenced the brain and when fresh blood has begun to flow through it on rewarming.

With his phalanx of specialists—cardiologists, anaesthetist, biochemists, metabolists, assistants and technicians—the modern heart surgeon has become only one man in a team which may number anything up to fifteen. And he would be first to agree that he and his knife would do little without the men around them.

9

Could we borrow another heart?

WORK on the heart-lung machine seemed to have come to a full stop when it suddenly regained its impetus through a discovery made by a British research doctor at the Royal College of Surgeons experimental farm in the South of England.

Anthony Andreasen and technician Frank Watson had gone back over shoals of medical literature asking themselves exactly how much blood the human body might need to keep both brain and body cells from perishing. William Harvey, in the seventeenth century, had answered part of the question by clamping off the hearts of snakes, watching them empty and re-fill and then continue to beat normally. For half a century surgeons had tried with the human heart and found they could deprive it of blood for several minutes. They noticed, too, that patients who had suffered serious haemorrhages appeared to manage well on very little blood.

All this background suggested to Andreasen that the flow of blood through the body might be reduced so that surgeons could by-pass the heart, open it and repair defects. To do this, he needed another circulation; and naturally he thought of a blood donor whose heart and lungs might serve the patient on the operating table.

The possibility of open-heart surgery had intrigued and attracted Andreasen for more than fifteen years before he started his experiments in 1950. As a student he had been struck by the techniques which the great French surgeon,

Alexis Carrel, had used to join blood vessels and transplant organs temporarily from one animal to another. Carrel's work first gave the young British surgeon the idea that perhaps he could establish a link between the circulation of two people and make it possible for one to take over the functions of the other while the heart was opened for surgery. In the Far East, where he worked from 1933 to 1947 with the Indian Medical Service, Andreasen had the opportunity to set up small laboratories to carry out experiments on blood circulation. As a surgeon with the Indian Army during the war, he saw many cases of heart wounds which seemed to bear out his theory that one heart might have the strength to support two human beings. Andreasen found himself in Calcutta as Professor of Surgery at the Medical College during the bloodbath which followed the partition of India, and had the opportunity to observe dozens of severe heart injuries.

Thrown out of the country when India became independent, Andreasen went to the United States with his ideas, but found little encouragement. In England, when he mooted his plans, the Royal College of Surgeons paid some attention, and with a £400-a-year grant from the Leverhulme Trust, he began in a small laboratory at the Buckston Browne experimental farm, at Downe, Kent, to put his theory to the tests. Watson, his collaborator, showed remarkable skill and ingenuity in rigging up the experimental apparatus out of bits and pieces. And, from next door, where a team from Hammersmith Hospital was devising a heart-lung machine, they received some help in analysing blood oxygen. The two experimenters, however, looked with a certain envy at the liberal financial help the Hammersmith team obtained—but they pressed on with their own string-and-sealing-wax work.

Andreasen turned to the Medical Research Council, Britain's official medical "Cabinet", for support with money and equipment. The M.R.C. sent one of their representatives to the

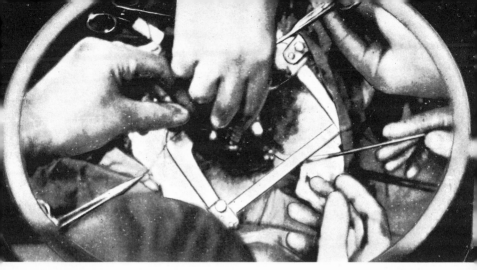

Below: The heart team from the Postgraduate Medical School at Hammersmith Hospital operating on a patient during their visit to Moscow in 1959. All four operations in which the surgeons stopped the heart to repair defects were successful. Above photograph shows a detail from a heart operation, illustrating how the ribs are retracted with a special instrument to expose the heart

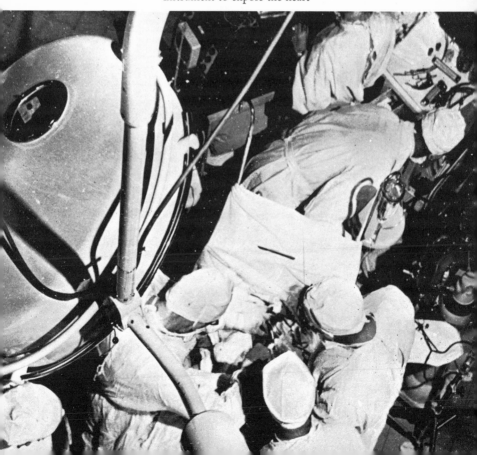

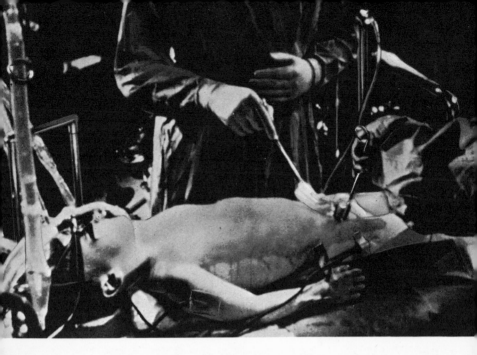

The boy on the operating table is clinically dead. By cooling his blood to 10° C. (50° F.),
surgeons have arrested his heart, his breathing and even the signals from his brain. *Below*,
a member of the operating team reads the "ticker tape" which monitors the heart beats,
brainwaves and temperatures while the boy is cooled

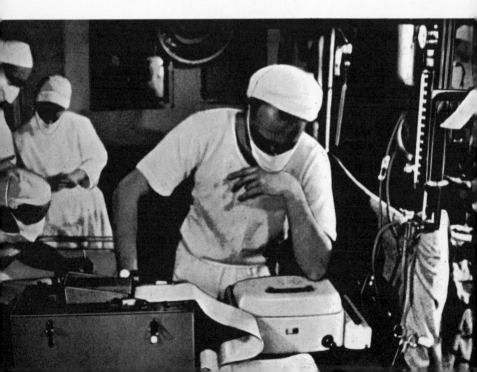

Buckston Browne farm to look over the research and talk to the two men. He glanced at the work, listened to their ideas and spent exactly seven minutes in their laboratory—they timed him. When he had run a civil service eye over the place he gave them the answer to their request for help in one word: "No." When they asked why, he said: "The day of the individual experimenter is over. It is teams of experts now."

Undeterred, Andreasen began to experiment with animals to see whether low blood flow would maintain life without injuring the organs. Sealing off the main veins to the heart and allowing blood to enter it from another vein, he found the critical survival flow to be between a tenth and a seventh of normal. From this, Andreasen inferred that one heart would support two lives while open-heart surgery was carried out. And so it proved on animals. Tying the major veins and arteries together and using a small, cheap pump to boost the circulation between donor and patient, the surgeon discovered he could keep both animals alive on a mere trickle of blood.

After dozens of animals had come unharmed through these cross-circulation experiments and operations, Andreasen went on to prove that this low blood flow would maintain life adequately while he isolated the heart from the circulation and carried out token surgical work. He came up with the same results—the animals could get by easily on a tenth of their normal blood ration.

Andreasen published his work in 1953. It raised no outcry, nor even enthusiasm. To most surgeons it seemed a nice piece of esoteric research, but where did it lead? Even heart surgeons skimmed over it, shoved it in their files and promptly forgot it.

Disillusioned and dejected, Andreasen decided to get out of Britain. He did not regret the fifteen years he had spent working on his theory, nor the five years it had taken him to confirm it—only the failure of his profession to appreciate the work and its implications. The British surgeon went abroad at the age of

48 to organize medical services for a mining company in Sierra Leone on the West African coast. Later he joined the Ghana medical service. As a final irony, Andreasen picked up a magazine in Africa—and saw that his research had at last been applied. There were pictures of operations in which his cross-circulation technique was saving lives.

For one surgeon had not spurned Andreasen's findings. At once he grasped the salient details of the British results and realized they meant the difference between success and failure, between allowing patients to die or giving them a chance to live. From Minneapolis, Dr. C. Walton Lillehei flew over to take a closer look at the British work. When he returned to the University of Minnesota Medical School he hustled his colleagues into a programme of research designed to confirm or refute Andreasen's work. Lillehei, Associated Professor of Surgery at Minnesota, is perhaps the most colourful figure heart surgery has thrown up. The son of a Norwegian dentist who settled in America, he had known surgery from both sides of the operating table. Two years before he began open-heart surgery he had himself recovered from a cancer operation. Controversy seemed to stick to him like a surgical glove to a hand. Some dismissed him as a young man in too much of a hurry; others described him as a genius. Everyone who knows him well agrees about one facet of his character: toughness and tenacity. With some surgeons, only published statistics matter and the life-or-death case which might spoil the record is hurriedly ducked. Not with Lillehei. If the surgeon can give the patient a chance, and he fails, it's just too bad about the figures—but the patient comes first.

Behind Lillehei stood a team of gifted surgeons, notably Herbert E. Warden, Richard L. Varco and Morley Cohen, who felt the same way. Soon this group had in its hands proof that animals could live on anything from a tenth to a seventh of their normal blood pressure. From a chance remark made by

Warden the idea of plugging one patient into the heart of another was born. The experiments with animals had worked; they had no reason to assume the same procedure would fail with human beings. The ethics of using a parent to transfuse blood into his child during an operation might worry the medical profession; it certainly would not upset the parent; nor did it matter greatly to the four doctors who agreed to stake their reputations on it.

As usual, their cases came from the lists of children who might not live long, and therefore had less chance of surviving major surgery. Their first patient was typical—a 12-month-old boy who had spent three-quarters of his life in hospital with recurrent heart failure and chest trouble. His father readily volunteered to lend his heart. So, on the 26th of March, 1954, came the dramatic moment when the father and son lay beside each other, lightly anaesthetized, while the surgeons worked to tie their circulations together. One team prepared the boy by opening his heart; the other made a small nick in the thigh of his father. Far into his leg artery and vein two long tubes were pushed and tied at the bottom to prevent the blood vessels collapsing. The other ends of the tubes were placed into the son's great veins and one of the arteries round the heart. To boost the circulation between father and son two small pumps were connected to the tubes and driven by an electric motor.

The system could hardly have worked better. For twelve and a half minutes the father supplied blood while the surgeons opened the right side of the heart. There they saw the hole which was killing the boy. A few minutes and several silk stitches later they had closed it. They congratulated themselves on two records: the first time that any surgeon had mended a hole in the main inside wall of the heart; and the first use of donor-circulation. The boy was well and looked as though he would leave hospital with a good heart.

But on the eleventh day, despite the improvement in his heart, he fell ill with pneumonia and died. To the statistician it might have spelled 100 per cent failure. The Minnesota team, however, knew the method worked. And the next two cases, both hole-in-the-heart children whose parents acted as donors, had their defects corrected with no complications during or after the operation.

Lillehei and his colleagues then went on to demonstrate that the most serious heart conditions could be tackled with cross circulation. These were the Blue Babies, who still relied on the Blalock-Taussig by-pass operation.

Alongside their first case in the hospital lay one of these children, an 11-year-old boy whom heart disease had crippled from birth. By now he could walk only one block before he had to rest on his haunches to regain his energy. The Minnesota surgeon who examined him in March concluded that he had little time to live if he did not have an operation. Heart soundings showed he had the classic series of defects making up the Tetralogy of Fallot—a blocked valve, ballooning right heart, a hole in the centre and a blood detour through the main artery.

Would the heart stand it? Would the donor method succeed? Could they hope to do a four-in-one operation? Courageously, on the 13th of August, 1954, the four surgeons linked up the boy and a 29-year-old donor from his home town who had volunteered to act as his heart. As they had feared, the weakened heart gave out, just at the moment they had placed the tube terminals in both patients. The top chambers of the boy's heart faltered and stopped, the bottom two quivered uselessly. The surgeons stopped for a moment to decide whether to massage the heart and then gave the order, "start the pumps". A few minutes later the heart took up its beat and kept on going placidly throughout the operation.

It was a Fallot, all right. High up between the two main

chambers of the heart they saw a hole a full inch and a quarter wide through which blood was sloshing. This, they closed, and then looked at the pulmonary valve, the three cusps of which had fused to close the opening to the lung arteries. They stretched the valve, and then closed the boy's chest. In fourteen days he had left the hospital; when he returned it was to tell the four surgeons about his baseball games and his cycling runs.

With their skill and determination, the Minnesota group had made open-heart surgery a reality. They proved that the first Blue-Baby operation had been no fluke when they ran off a whole series. Perhaps the most curious of the forty-six operations they performed with the help of donors took place on the 6th of May, 1955. The heart cripple was a boy of 10 who had the usual history—but complicated with heart block, a condition where the top and bottom chambers beat out of phase with distressing results.

A friend of the boy's family agreed to act as donor. But before this man of 31 could help with his circulation the boy's heart began to play tricks, racing when the surgeons touched it and beating irregularly. Painstakingly, the surgeons plugged their tube sockets into the vessels surrounding the heart, but even this gentle handling sent the heart fluttering until finally it all but came to a standstill. Only the starting of the donor's circulation brought the heartbeat back into its regular rhythm.

The hole in the centre of the heart was big, just under two inches. But the surgeons had little difficulty bringing its ragged ends together. The blocked valve gave them no trouble. However, as they repaired the two defects they saw something else—through the three-leaved valve beating between the right upper and lower chambers of the heart appeared another hole! So twice they had to open the heart and make good the three-quarter-inch tear between the atria. The boy recovered and had a new heart.

As a surgical *tour de force*, the donor-circulation series in those two years bear comparison with anything in the history of heart operations. Lillehei was not only able to point to the success of the method; his statistics satisfied even the most highly critical of his rivals.

But cross-circulation raised far too many moral as well as technical problems. Surgeons in Britain and America shied away from the thought of confronting parents with the Hobson's Choice of acting as a second heart in operations on their children.

Gibbon, whose machine had by now been adopted by the Mayo Clinic and would shortly prove successful, expressed himself forcibly on this point when Lillehei revealed that he had carried out these parent-and-child operations. In reply to Lillehei, Gibbon told the congress of the American Association for Thoracic Surgery in Montreal: "We are still convinced that it is preferable to perform operations involving open cardiotomy by some procedure which does not involve another healthy person. There must be some risk to the donor in a cross circulation."

Lillehei had proved to his own satisfaction that little or no risk existed; but he took the hint, and his team at Minneapolis began to look for alternatives. Two of his collaborators, Dr. Gilbert S. Campbell and Dr. Norman W. Crisp, hit on the idea of trying animal lungs to keep the blood fresh.

Before them lay the results of experimental work by a group of Canadian surgeons, led by Dr. William Mustard, who had verified that the lungs of monkeys could serve as a stand-in for human lungs. The two Americans soon went to Lillehei with proof that dog lungs, sterilized and prepared, would act as the vital oxygenator. Soon, the surgeons confirmed the lab. work by carrying out the first operation; then followed fourteen others with the biological oxygenator.

But, again, this method lent itself to criticism, and while it saved lives, the surgeons knew they had to resolve the problem of aerating the blood with a more permanent apparatus. Hand-in-hand with the research on cross-circulation and animal lungs, the quest had gone on for a heart-lung machine which would deliver enough oxygen to the blood. At Minneapolis they decided that Gibbon, with his complicated and expensive equipment, had not found the answer; nor had the Swedes, who had designed a workable pump as far back as 1946.

Early in 1954, Lillehei handed the problem to a former family doctor, now one of his young laboratory research workers. Richard A. De Wall thought he might produce a mechanical lung by injecting large oxygen bubbles into a tall tube of blood. It sounded easy; but De Wall and Lillehei well knew that bubbles in the blood stream were worse than heart disease; they could cause a fatal airlock and had to be removed as soon as enough oxygen had adhered to the blood. De Wall's large-bubble theory worked; the oxygen saturation of blood pleased both physicians and surgeons. But look at a glass of soda water and you will get some impression of the difficulty which the research man faced when he came to remove the countless bubbles from blood. He solved it ingeniously by placing an anti-bubbling chamber at the top of his tall mixing tube. In this chamber, sponges of stainless steel coated with an anti-foam chemical broke up the bubbles of oxygen and allowed them to escape through a vent at the top. This accounted for large bubbles; to filter out the small bubbles De Wall fashioned several feet of plastic tubing in a helter-skelter shape through which the blood spiralled downwards after it left the debubbler. The bubble problem beaten, De Wall made light work of the machine, which he completed in not much more than a year.

The finished machine, its parts made of smooth stainless steel and plastic, soon established itself in laboratory trials. It worked thus: the three tubes were connected to the great veins and a main artery. A pump impelled the spent venous blood into the bubble chamber where oxygen revitalized it and forced it to give up waste carbon dioxide. Both oxygen bubbles and the carbon dioxide were removed in the debubbling compartment before the blood fell into the plastic coil. A water bath at body temperature kept the blood warm before a second pump took over to drive it back into the patient's body through an artery, either near the heart or in the thigh. The Lillehei-De Wall machine appealed to surgeons. It was cheap, simple, efficient and soon found its way into the research departments of many hospitals which were building up teams for heart surgery.

But a few months before Lillehei felt ready to operate with his machine another group of doctors in the same State announced they had done four successful open-heart operations with Gibbon's heart-lung apparatus. The Mayo Clinic, first in so many medical fields, had finally proved that the Gibbon machine had needed no more than a team of good surgeons round it to redeem it from the laboratory workshop. Dr. John W. Kirklin, and seven colleagues, did eight open-heart cases and pronounced their faith in the machine; it merely required practice, like all other surgery.

The Gibbon and Lillehei machines revolutionized heart surgery in the United States. And at the same time, in Britain, surgeons had not remained idle, and were now ready to keep pace with their American colleagues.

10

The First Stopped-Heart Operation

ONE OTHER person was watching the work which Andreasen had done to prove the low-flow principle —a young Oxford graduate who worked at the Buckston Browne farm side by side with the surgeon. But Denis Melrose had other ideas, among them the determination to build a machine which would short-circuit the heart and make open-heart operations routine.

Melrose had come to the Postgraduate Medical School at Hammersmith in 1949. At that time the school had decided to carry out a programme of basic research on cancer, using pumps to circulate blood and oxygen through cancerous organs removed at operations to test response to anti-cancer drugs. The dark-haired assistant lecturer followed the instructions of his head of department, Professor Ian Aird, and set up apparatus for these perfusion experiments.

But, secretly, Melrose had become a disciple of Gibbon, and realized that, though the heart-lung machine might have a few "bugs" in it, there was nothing which modifications would not fix. So, in addition to his cancer experiments, Melrose began to plan the first British heart-lung machine. He went to the literature, and there found papers by a Swedish surgeon that many research minds had missed. The Swedes had, indeed, achieved as much success as Gibbon in a different field.

The same Clarence Crafoord who sectioned and joined the first constricted aorta, had followed up his work. Two years after this operation he had, with an engineer, built a machine to fulfil the functions of the heart and lungs. Crafoord's idea did not extend to the complete isolation of the heart. Before his famous operation he had proved that the main blood trunk could be clamped off for thirty minutes without damaging the major internal organs. But the brain cells, ultra-sensitive to oxygen starvation, begin to perish irrevocably in three minutes. If he could find a way of keeping the brain alive, then the heart could be taken out of the body circulation, opened and repaired.

The machine which Crafoord and his associate designed and constructed appeared crude by present standards. But it possessed the essential elements of the modern heart-lung apparatus; it lacked only engineering finesse. The important thing was that it worked. Faced with the problem of recharging blood with oxygen, the Swedes had replaced Gibbon's mesh screens with a revolving drum of transparent plastic. Fifty large stainless-steel discs inside the drum collected the blood flowing through it while oxygen was blown along its axis against the flow. A special compressed-air pump drove the blood round the circuit. To avoid damaging the blood the pump acted like a vice, squeezing the blood through the circuit.

Another surgeon at the Sabbatsberg Hospital began experimenting with animals, using Crafoord's machine as soon as it had been tested. Viking Olov Björk, one of the pioneers of modern heart-lung surgery, wondered if he could keep the brain, the most vital part of the body, alive while he cut off the circulation to the heart. He tapped into the main artery and vein leading through the neck to the brain, plugged these blood vessels into the machine and set it going. Then he sealed off the great veins which drain all the blood from the body into the right chambers of the heart. Slowly the heart emptied— and Björk counted thirty-three minutes before releasing the clamps from the veins.

In 1948, the Swedish surgeon could report not one failure.

Neither brain nor body had suffered. The great work of Crafoord and Björk had opened the way to the surgery of defects on the right side of the heart. The Swedes had shown, too, that machines might either assist the blood circulation, keep certain parts of the body alive while surgeons operate elsewhere, or even act as heart and lungs.

British surgeons were impressed. Melrose paid a visit to Stockholm a year after Björk's paper had appeared and looked closely at the Crafoord machine and the experiments the Sabbatsberg staff had done with it. The young British surgeon acknowledged his debt to the Swedes when his own machine made its appearance.

At first, surgeons in the Postgraduate Medical School viewed these robots not as a means of by-passing the heart to allow it to be bared for surgery; they inclined to treat them more as a booster to a failing heart and circulation during operations. But they gave Melrose a free hand to build his machine, and soon he and three of his hospital colleagues were working with outside designers to improve on the Gibbon and Swedish designs.

They leaned more towards Crafoord's machine. The finished version had, as its central piece, a rotating plastic cyclinder canted slightly to allow blood to run through unassisted. The 30-inch cyclinder was packed with seventy-six discs and washers. Melrose contended that the blood should be filmed on to the plates for at least half a second to pick up oxygen and release its carbon dioxide. And there should, he emphasized, be no foaming of blood. Ingeniously, the designers hit on the idea of giving the discs and the washers a contrary movement inside the drum so that the blood did not pile up on the bottom. This meant the machine needed less blood to prime it—a problem with American and Swedish types. The oxygen was blown through the cylinder against the blood flow through it. Everyone agreed that the Hammersmith apparatus seemed a beautiful piece of precision engineering. Would it work in practice?

At Buckston Browne in 1953 a team of surgeons from the hospital tried it out on animals. They did no heart operations, only experiments to see if the machine could assist the circulation. It behaved as well as it looked: the team declared it ready for the operating theatre.

The machine had its baptism on a cold December afternoon in 1953 when it helped to save the life of a woman stricken with heart trouble. The physicians and surgeons who had examined the woman decided she would have little chance of surviving a normal heart operation, and had, in fact, ruled out an operation for acute appendix some months before because she was too grave a risk. The diagnosis pointed to mitral and aortic valve disease.

The team, Ian Aird, William Cleland, Melrose and Dr. Beverley Lynn made no attempt to exclude the heart. Instead they opened the main artery and vein in the right thigh and tapped these with the input and output tubes of the machine. Then, as the pumps began to push about one pint of blood a minute into the artery, Cleland, the surgeon, approached the heart from the left side. When he probed through an incision in the left auricle he found the two leaves of the mitral valve were retracted rather than fused.

The pumps stepped up their output as the surgeon opened the left chamber of the heart. Through this wound he explored the three-leaved valve at the entrance to the aorta and discovered this to be constricted. With a special instrument he stretched the valve three times. Throughout the operation the heart rhythm remained steady. Tests, made after the surgeons had closed the chest, revealed no changes in the blood or the brain. The machine had come through its first trial; now the hospital began to build up a team around Cleland, which has become famous wherever heart specialists gather. But, at first the

Hammersmith staff learned the technique slowly and methodically, contenting themselves with the minor defects of the
heart. Melrose, however, was working on something which,
used with his machine, might completely change the face of
heart surgery. Nothing less than the stopping of the heart itself.
During open-heart surgery with the Gibbon and Lillehei
techniques the heart still functioned, fed by the blood draining
into the coronary arteries and veins supplying its own muscle.
Surgeons might open the heart and draw off this blood; but
the organ still pulsing at seventy or more beats a minute proved
tricky and slippery to handle. Especially where a whole series
of defects had to be found and corrected in the shortest time.
The beating heart presented another problem: air lock. Closing
the heart and allowing it to fill with blood after an operation
might leave air in one of its compartments, and an air bubble
driven round the circulation might dam the flow of blood
and cause death. Sucking air out of the heart as it refilled, or
syphoning off the air—these were the manœuvres which open-
heart surgeons were then using.

To give surgeons a clear, unhurried look at the heart,
Melrose began with three colleagues to try stopping and restarting the hearts of animals coupled to the machine. The
medical literature was encouraging. Sydney Ringer, the great
English physician, had shown in 1883 that various chemical
substances affected the heart beat. In America two surgeons
had more recently studied the effect of potassium chloride on
the heart. In experiments to stop and revive the heart the
Hammersmith group could not endorse the American work.

Instead they began a series of experiments which lasted more
than two years. First, they used isolated hearts kept alive on a
system of tubes, and on these they tested the effect of potassium
citrate. Then they kept animals alive with the Melrose machine
while they duplicated these experiments.

When the machine had taken over the functions of the

heart and lungs the surgeons clamped off the major veins and the main arteries to allow the heart to empty. Then beneath the aorta clamp they injected a solution of potassium citrate. In a few seconds the heart began to beat slowly; in five seconds it had become a limp, flaccid organ. A token operation was performed. The surgeons found that, in its limp state, they could easily expel the air from the heart before closing the operation wound. They observed, too, that it remained pink and healthy throughout the procedure.

For fifteen minutes they kept hearts at a standstill. Then, by releasing the clamps and letting the blood flow back into the arteries they watched them pick up and start beating. Sometimes they had to help the organ along with drugs, but when it started the muscle tone seemed good.

They appeared to have beaten the problem—with one big BUT: no sooner had the heart resumed its beat than it turned into a squirming, wriggling mass. This fibrillation often stops when the heart is given a slight shock, but in only seven cases out of ten did the shock stir the heart into its normal rhythm. To the Hammersmith research group it meant going back to basic work all over again.

Carefully they checked over their previous experiments using varying doses of potassium citrate and observing the effects on stopping and restarting the heart. Their original idea had been sound; the doses of chemical had merely been too great. Smaller amounts brought about heart arrest equally effectively, but made it easier to restore the heart beat.

Now they had satisfied themselves. The team, in their publication of the results, said much work required to be done on heart arrest, but their research proved that the stop-heart technique would make surgery possible in a dry, limp heart without the danger of airlock in the bloodstream.

The Hammersmith report appeared in July, 1955. But the surgeons in the London teaching centre did not have the opportunity to confirm their research successes in the operating theatre. Such was the pace of cardiac surgery that at that time the work in Hammersmith inspired several American centres to carry out similar experiments.

In Cleveland, Ohio, a group of doctors had studied the Melrose paper with more than ordinary interest. One of these, a tall, bespectacled Dutchman, had worked for some time at Hammersmith Hospital and knew the men who had experimented with heart arrest. Dr. Willem Kolff was that rare combination, a doctor who had a genius with the mind and hands for biological engineering. Kolff, who seriously thinks that most parts of the body might be fashioned in the laboratory, had in Holland during the war, under the eyes of the Nazis, built and smuggled out the first crude artificial kidney—from nothing more than a few bits of metal, sausage skins and a beer barrel. He bequeathed this machine to Hammersmith when he left for America.

Immediately he read the Hammersmith report, Kolff, Dr. Donald Effler and members of the research division of the Cleveland Clinic Foundation set to work experimentally. In six months they had confirmed the Hammersmith work. The next month they felt ready to try it out on one of the many patients who waited with hole-in-the-heart trouble.

First on their list came a thin, dark-haired child of 17 months. Heart soundings with the tube-in-the-vein technique disclosed a hole in his heart between the two main chambers. They decided to try Melrose's method of arresting his heart, and set the operation date for the 17th of February, 1956.

On the 16th of February Melrose was working in the Postgraduate Medical School at Hammersmith Hospital when the call came through from Cleveland. He picked up the telephone for what must rank as one of the most expensive consultations ever held. Kolff was on the other end of the line. Briefly he explained that they had been working on stopped-heart experiments: now they wanted to tackle the case of a child seriously ill with a heart defect. Could the British surgeon run over the technique he had used, and any new data which he had discovered in the last seven months? For more than half an hour Melrose explained the methods he and his collaborators had used, and how he would employ these in the operating theatre. The Dutchman listened, took notes of the details and went back to tell Dr. Effler that the operation was on.

The American surgeons used Kolff's heart-lung machine built on his string-and-sealing wax principle. While the Mayo Clinic worked with the costly Gibbon apparatus, and other hospitals had not stinted themselves on costs, Kolff had constructed his apparatus for not much more than £5. Its core consisted of a large tin can wrapped in twenty-two feet of plastic tubing with a plastic refrigerator as its jacket. Through the tubing which breathes but does not leak a small pump pours blood which receives pure oxygen as it flows.

The Cleveland surgeons, prompted by Melrose, gave themselves only fifteen minutes inside the empty and motionless heart. Anything longer than fifteen minutes and they knew the heart might rebel against resuming its beat.

Effler quickly exposed the child's heart, small and beating rapidly. Two leads from the machine were plugged through the upper chamber of the heart into the great veins; a third went into one of the branches of the main blood vessel. While they prepared the machine to take the strain off the heart, the surgeon measured out two thimblefuls of a clear fluid, potassium citrate, and charged his syringe with it. Then blood, treated with an anti-clotting drug, was used to dilute the potassium in the hypodermic.

As Kolff switched on the machine to maintain the circulation the heart of the child shrank, but still beat. The main artery was then drawn forward and clamped just above the point where it left the heart.

An X-ray picture of a pacemaker which has been sewn under the skin of an elderly man suffering from heart block. The size and shape of a pocket-watch, this small, battery-driven apparatus will feed impulses of a few volts into the heart muscles to keep the organ beating at about sixty times a second. This type of pacemaker is recharged by induction from a power source placed just outside the chest. *Below*, another form of pacemaker which is connected to a battery carried by the patient

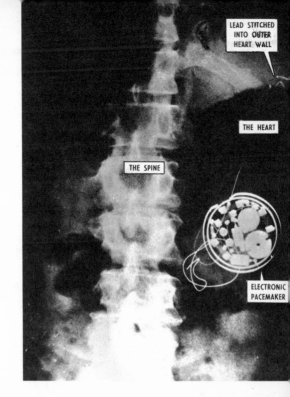

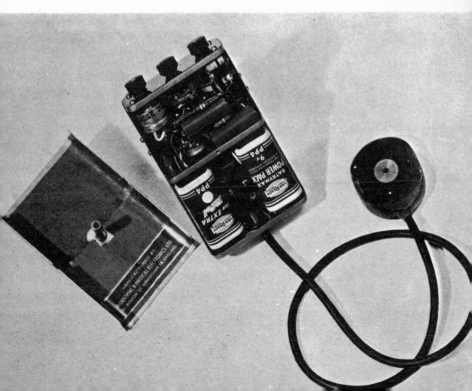

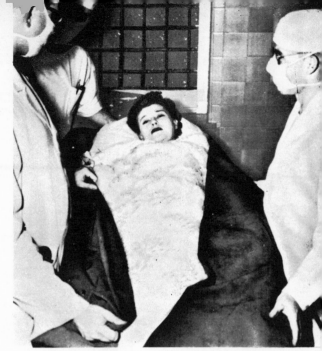

Doctors at the Michael Reese Hospital, Chicago, demonstrate a method of cooling for heart operations. The patient is packed in shaved ice until her temperature drops to 79° F. and the heart can be opened without endangering her life

A patient in a British hospital where another method of surface cooling is used. The body is immersed in a household bath of iced water to bring down the temperature to just over 80° F. Hands and feet are kept out of the water to prevent frostbite

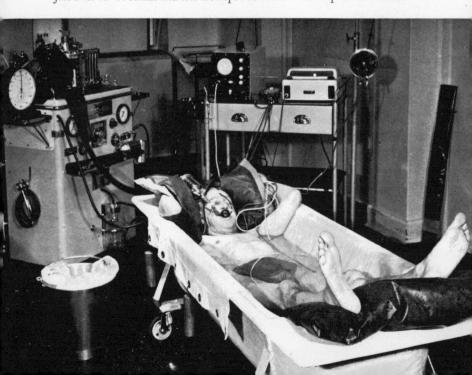

The time was noted. Dr. Effler then pierced the main artery with the syringe needle—guarded by a plastic collar to prevent him going too deep—and rapidly emptied it watching the heart action as he pressed the plunger. As the chemical found its way into the coronary arteries, the heart began to pulse more slowly. Within seconds the two main pumping chambers had stopped; then the auricles, until only the tip of the right auricle seemed to quiver. The heart had stopped—they had fifteen minutes now to repair it as it lay, dead, looking larger than ever, in its chest niche.

Thirteen minutes were all Effler needed. Deftly he placed stay stitches along the right ventricle to hold open the wound, and then made his incision. Normally, with a beating heart the hole in its main inside wall would have gaped open like a large coin; now it lay like a frayed button-hole in the still heart. It took a matter of minutes to pull it together with silk thread, reinforcing the edges with more stitches. The surgeons found time to inspect the pulmonary valve and the upper heart chambers before closing the wound.

The heart had stopped readily enough. Would it start again? Effler, following Melrose's technique, released the clamp over the main artery to allow blood to flush into the heart arteries. As this blood washed the potassium mixture out of the arteries the heart began to move. In a few seconds it was beating as though it had never stopped.

Fourteen days after the operation the child whose heart had been "dead" and restored to life, was walking around the ward of the clinic; eight months later a plump-faced, bow-tied child appeared again at the hospital for re-examination. His heart, once crippled, was now normal in every way.

Of course, several surgeons cribbed at the idea of stopping the most vital of all the functions—the heart beat. Some objected that it might increase heart block, a dangerous condition in which the upper and lower chambers of the heart beat out of phase; the stitches, some contended, had to be placed in the beating heart so that defects could be repaired correctly.

The Cleveland team answered these objections with a run of 73 stopped-heart operations in fifteen months, and no more than the usual mortality. In May, 1957, Effler was able to tell the American Association for Thoracic Surgery at Chicago: "On the basis of this experience, a preliminary conclusion is justified, namely: The safety and the benefits provided by the Melrose technique for elective cardiac arrest justify its use in surgery on the open heart."

II

Invitation to Moscow

THE HOSPITAL which wanted to specialize in open-heart surgery needed a well-tried machine. Around this they had to drill a well-knit unit of surgeons, cardiologists and doctors who understood the machine. The Gibbon episode had amply proved this. His heart-lung apparatus was little better when it came out of the laboratory for the second time; but the Mayo team had welded it into their brilliant technique to make a success of open-heart operations. So it happened in other hospitals which used machines for the first time, even with the poor-risk patients which they were given when other treatments had failed. Some surgeons were shocked by the high mortality and a number gave up; but the far-sighted struggled on, profiting by their errors and finding that skill and experience could reduce the death-rate to somewhere around six in every hundred patients.

At the Postgraduate Medical School in Hammersmith, William Cleland had gathered a gifted group of surgeons round the Melrose machine. He was lucky to have in the school one of the best cardiologists in the country, Dr. John Goodwin, and his assistant, Dr. Arthur Hollman. The surgeon who operates without adequate briefing by his heart specialist often has to cope with emergencies which might have been foreseen in reading the results of cardiograms, catheterization, or in ordinary diagnosis.

The Hammersmith team consisted of no less than twelve surgeons and doctors, each of them doing a vital job during heart operations. Around Cleland, a stocky, good-humoured Australian and a brilliant chest surgeon, the hospital built the team into one of the finest in the world. They studied and rehearsed each operation until it was a piece of meticulous discipline.

Within a couple of years of the first baptism of the Melrose machine they had worked their way through dozens of hole-in-the-heart cases with a very low death-rate. Notable among them was a fair-haired, bright boy of seven who seemed an ordinary case—until they opened his heart.

The diagnosis told them that the boy had a tear in the main heart wall; only the peculiar shape of the heart wave on the electrocardiogram suggested something strange.

But when Cleland made a slit in the right ventricle he found the boy had only one lower chamber; the dividing tissue had gone completely. The surgeons had to make a plastic patch about one and a half inches long by just over an inch wide and stitch it into the ventricle to create a new septum.

The Hammersmith team had done dozens of open-heart operations when a request came from Russia for one of the new Melrose heart-lung units in the country. The makers, New Electronic Products Ltd., sent a machine to Moscow.

Russian surgeons had accomplished much during the war in heart surgery; but none had ever used a machine to short-circuit the heart; nor had they kept in close touch with American and British experience. They tried the Melrose machine experimentally and came back to the British surgeons saying, "This machine does not work."

Technicians flew to Russia, took the machine apart and assured the Soviet surgeons that mechanically it was perfect. Again the Russians tried; and once more they failed with their open-heart experiments. Through the Russian Embassy in London, Professor Bakulev, President of the U.S.S.R. Academy of Medical Sciences, made an approach to the

Department of Surgery at Hammersmith. Would a team of British surgeons care to visit Moscow and stage a series of operations on Russian children for the benefit of their medical leaders?

Hammersmith immediately replied, "Yes." It was an invitation unprecedented in surgical history. Not since Peter the Great bought a whole anatomical museum in Holland at the beginning of the eighteenth century and shipped it to Russia had such a request been made. It meant virtually transferring the whole surgical theatre to Moscow—everything from the machine and the men, to instruments, the linen suturing materials and curved needles. Naturally, the invitation caused misgivings. Mortality still remained a big factor in all heart operations; the team would carry out their work in a blaze of world publicity; in a strange theatre watched by an eminent audience; and with the possibility that some of their patients might die on the table or following the operations. There was even the unanswered question about the patients. Obviously they would be chosen from poor-risk heart cases, since the Russians knew little or nothing about the open-heart technique. What if one of them were the son or daughter of some Communist big-wig?

With him, Cleland took Melrose and surgeon Hugh Bentall, anaesthetist John Beard, cardiologist Arthur Hollman and technician John Robson. The only woman in the party was theatre sister Phyllis Bowtle. On the 23rd of April, 1959, they sailed in the Russian ship *Baltika* for Leningrad and there put their gear on the train for Moscow.

Cleland and Hollman looked over the cases carefully. Each one of the four girls who were chosen from dozens at the Moscow Institute of Thoracic Surgery was catheterized by the young, fair-haired Hammersmith cardiologist: traces were taken of their hearts, and the various other clinical tests completed. Two of them were Blue Babies; another had a hole in the heart between the lower chambers; and the fourth had a tear between the two receiving compartments.

The British surgeons were treated with typical Russian hospitality as they made the ward rounds in the Moscow hospital. They answered hundreds of questions about their stopped-heart method; about the machine; and about the fifty cases they had done in England.

In the morning of the 11th of May they did the first of their big operations. Behind the glass wall of the observation gallery crowded surgeons from Leningrad, Moscow and other Soviet centres. In the theatre were Bakulev and the medical director of the Moscow Institute, Professor Mikhail Tsentsiper, with the interpreter who described the details of the operation. And, rare in Britain, unheard of in Russia, were photographers from the Russian agency, Tass, to record scenes from the operation.

The patient, a quiet, six-year-old Russian girl called Lucia Demecheva, was brought into the theatre and placed on the table near the heart-lung machine, and the three-hour operation had begun.

The Russian surgeons took notes of everything. They watched Beard anaesthetizing the girl with a barbiturate injection into an arm vein; then the later administration of curare through the same vein to relax the muscles. One of their own anaesthetists took over the breathing with artificial respiration through an air bladder as the surgeons slipped a tube tip into the left arm vein to give blood when they felt it necessary. Next, a catheter was slipped through a right arm vein deep into a main heart vein to measure blood pressure and to give fluids during the operation.

Cleland now made a deep incision down the line of the breastbone and behind this slipped a slender, pliable saw to divide the bone which was then drawn back with rib retractors. He opened the pericardium and pulled back the edges of this heart sac to expose the heart. Before the surgeon could start linking the machine to the Russian girl he had to search for defects which might hamper the flow from the machine through the body. An open duct between the pulmonary and main artery would have to be tied off. He found none—and the surgeons began quickly and methodically to work round the pounding heart, isolating it and leading the plastic artery and vein from the machine which had been charged with blood.

The aorta, the main from the heart, was freed to make clamping easier when the time came. A cut-down laid open an artery in the thigh which would take the fresh blood passing through the mechanical pump. And last of all, two nicks were made in the upper right chamber of the heart and through these two nozzles from the outflow line were placed into the main veins.

The pump was then switched on and for a few minutes the surgeons allowed it to assist the heart, before tightening the snares on the pump lines tied into the vessels round the heart. As the heart was isolated, and the pump took over its work, the four chambers of the heart seemed to sag and shrink. Through its right ventricle a sucker was passed to empty the blood which continued to flow into the heart from its own network of veins and the lungs.

Now came the dramatic highlight of the operation. The Russians watched eagerly as Cleland took a syringe with a needle no more than a third of an inch long. The aorta was clamped and into a point just beneath the clamp the surgeon squirted the potassium citrate and blood mixture which caused the heart to flag and collapse in a few seconds. Carefully the hole in the artery was stitched—and the main part of the operation began.

Cleland opened the right ventricle with a long incision which gave him a clear sight of the inside of the heart. High up in the heart wall was the defect through which blood sloshed; and beside it lay the blocked pulmonary valve which hampered the outflow of blood to the lungs. A sucker was run across the edges of the hole to help the surgeon map its extent and decide whether or not he needed a plastic patch. The valve was also explored before the surgeon turned to the defect. He had half an hour to make good the faults before the heart should be restarted, for anything over this period might make things difficult.

The job called for care. Stitches placed hurriedly might damage the aortic valve near the hole; they might, too, upset the heart muscle which regulates its beat. So each thread was sited carefully though quickly and tied separately. To allow the heart to accustom itself to the sealing of the hole, a small gap was left while the surgeon opened the fused valve cusps.

The heart was closed by suturing the incision, leaving a sucker inside to flush out the heart through the right ventricle, then the surgeon released the clamp on the main artery to allow blood to run into the heart and wash out the chemical which had stopped it. Within two to three minutes the heart began to beat, slowly at first and then more powerfully. The sucker was withdrawn and the ventricle closed. Now the pump and oxygenator which had maintained the circulation gradually gave place to the heart, the chest was closed and the tubes withdrawn from the blood vessels. The operation was over.

The heart had ceased to beat for twenty-five minutes while they fixed its defects. Now, when the surgeons had satisfied themselves it was beating regularly again, the girl was wheeled out of the theatre and placed in an oxygen tent in a ward to be nursed continuously for the first twenty-four hours, and carefully afterwards to see how the rest of her body stood up to the more powerful heart action. For two days after the operation, the girl showed the strain, and then started to get better.

A week later when she sat up and talked to her friends visiting the hospital, this Blue Baby told them, "I shall dance . . . I say it to myself every minute . . . I shall be able to dance."

The Hammersmith team carried through three more success-ful operations. They repaired heart defects in Yrena Belkova, aged 12, Gallina Skopkena, and Marie Ravechevskaya, both aged seven.

The operations, reported at length in *Pravda* and *Izvestia*, caught the imagination of the Russian public and the Kremlin leaders. The surgeons were fêted wherever they went.

On the 16th of May, when a Russian TU 104 jet brought them into London Airport, there, waiting with colleagues from Hammersmith Hospital was a familiar figure, slim and distinguished, to greet them and congratulate them on their success. It was Dr. John Gibbon, the pioneer of the heart-lung machine.

12

The Man in the Coffin

THE HEART-LUNG machine still sat as an unfulfilled blueprint when surgeons began to cast around for other methods of protecting the brain and the body during heart operations. Through the medical literature they found clues going as far back as 1756 which gave them the solution to heart surgery in one word: Hypothermia.

The medical meaning of hypothermia is the lowering of the body temperature by artificial means. Cooling the body meant that its cells would demand less oxygen and less nourishment. Did not hibernating animals prove this? And, could cooling not therefore protect the ultra-sensitive brain cells and other organs during surgery?

These thoughts began to excite the interest of surgeons just after the war. Thumbing through the literature, many research workers and surgeons raised their eyebrows on discovering that hypothermia had a long history.

An apochrypha of tales existed about ice-age mammoths and other animals reviving when they were dug up, aeons old, in odd parts of the world. The first authenticated record appears in the proceedings of the Swedish Academy of Sciences in 1757.

This was the case of the Swede whose relatives nearly buried him alive. This peasant, who had drunk too much brandy, was bowled over by a strong wind on the 23rd of March, 1756, collapsed in the snow and fell asleep. Uncovered the next morning, his relatives put him in a coffin and prepared to bury him. But before they could carry out the interment, their doctor, Sven Naucler, arrived unexpectedly and asked to examine the body.

The face, hands and feet were frozen, their joints locked with the cold, the eyes were fixed and staring, the heart still and the breathing arrested. But Dr. Naucler thought he detected a small region of warmth at the pit of the stomach. He ordered the man's legs and arms to be rubbed while he placed hot towels on the stomach. To their general astonishment, the man gradually stirred, later sat up, and by the next day was recovering.

Two more eighteenth-century surgeons believed in the virtues of cold. Dr. James Currie, an eminent and observant Liverpool surgeon, wondered what killed sailors who were shipwrecked in the Mersey. In 1798 he persuaded people to take prolonged baths in cold water and noted their temperature and pulse. As their body lost heat, Currie found the heart rate also flagged. Curiously enough, the chilly volunteers grew colder when they came out of the water; and more surprisingly when they were dipped into water at normal body temperature—98.4 degrees, Fahrenheit. Currie believed that he could evolve a treatment for fever based on hot and cold baths.

John Hunter, surgeon, anatomist, zoologist and body-snatcher, also left a legacy of hypothermia experiments. A visionary whose dreams were founded on experimental and scientific logic, Hunter imagined he might use deep-freeze treatment to prolong life.

Intrigued by the stories he had heard of fish and snakes reviving after being frozen, Hunter, the inveterate experimenter, did a series of scientific tests on animals at his private zoo in Earls Court, London, during January, 1777. Watched by two Glasgow University lecturers, Hunter prepared a tub of ice and then placed two carp in it. They died when he tried to resuscitate them; so did a couple of dormice, snails and other animals. In his lectures on the principles of surgery, Hunter mentions the experiments, and adds: "Till this time I had imagined that it might be possible to prolong life to any period by freezing a person in the frigid zone, as I thought all action and waste would cease till the body thawed. I thought that, if a man would give up the last ten years of his life to this kind of alternate oblivion and action, it might be prolonged to a thousand years; and by getting himself thawed every hundred years, he might learn what had happened during his frozen condition."

"Like other schemers," Hunter remarks sardonically, "I thought I should make my fortune by it; but this experiment undeceived me." Many a hard-headed surgeon would say today that Hunter's methods might have misled him, but his vision, as in so many other matters, was clear.

The retreat from Moscow introduced many stories of surgeons amputating frostbitten legs, or piling snow on limbs to reduce their circulation and their feeling before performing amputation. Napoleon's brilliant and resourceful surgeon, Baron Larrey, performed many amputations during the long walk back from Moscow by using snow or ice as both a local anaesthetic and to staunch the haemorrhage from surgical wounds.

But hypothermia as a medical remedy remained on the shelf for 140 years before two American doctors considered using it to treat cases with inoperable cancer. In 1938, Temple Fay and Laurence Smith, of Philadelphia, began to ask themselves why body cancers rarely spread to the limbs. They thought it might have something to do with the fact that the extremities are anything from six to twenty degrees colder than the trunk. Cancers, they knew, have a higher temperature than surrounding tissue. Fay and Smith reasoned that by dropping the body temperature they might halt or slow the growths. They took hopeless cancer cases and cooled them with ice packs down to 80 degrees—18 below normal—and kept the patients in this frozen-sleep state for eight days. The doctors were wrong: hypothermia had no effect on the tumours, but it did ease the pain over long periods and reduced their patients' dependence on pain-killing drugs. Fay and Smith, however, had broken the long clinical calm on hypothermia. Their report, in 1940, renewed the interest of doctors and surgeons in other applications of cold sleep.

The year when hypothermia began to mean something in medical literature was 1950. Not surprisingly, the first breakthrough came from Canada, with its extensive Arctic frontier and profound interest in the effects of cold. The Canadian Defence Board had given one of their most talented surgeons a grant to carry out experiments on how the body might react to intense cold.

Professor Wilfred G. Bigelow and two of his associates spent two years in the laboratory and then printed a report which proved that hypothermia could become a tool for the general surgeon. Bigelow cooled animals by wrapping them in special blankets through which he ran ice-cold spirit. Down to 64 degrees Fahrenheit he took the animals, watching the heart and brain activity and other reactions. At that temperature the heart beat had slowed from its upper limit of 180 to about 25 beats a minute; the animals were anaesthetized by the cold; their breathing and other body requirements had fallen. No animal suffered ill-effects from the cooling and the token operations which the Canadian performed. Bigelow realized the importance of the research. It abolished the need for the heroic "blind" methods of operating on the valves of the heart; and it allowed access to the inside of the organ for long enough to patch the less complicated defects.

His report opened with this passage which inspired so much later study of surgery using hypothermia:

"The use of hypothermia as a form of anaesthetic may conceivably extend the scope of surgery in many new directions. A state in which the body temperature is lowered and the oxygen requirements to tissues are reduced to a small fraction of normal would allow exclusion of organs from the circulation for prolonged periods. Such a technique may permit surgeons to operate on a bloodless heart without recourse to extracorporal pumps, and perhaps allow transplantation of organs."

Bigelow's report incited surgeons and physicians all over the world to study the way in which temperature reduction affected the body; it inspired a closer look at the hibernating animals to see if man could not borrow some of their tricks and perform them in the operating theatre.

Research soon pointed to deep distinctions between hibernation and hypothermia. Animals like the squirrel, the hamster and the dormouse, birds such as bats, all have some inner physiological mechanism which pulls down their heart beat, breathing and then their temperature to something close to that of surrounding conditions. Human beings have no such facility and keep a constant temperature, within small variations, however cold or hot their environment.

Animals, however, had much to teach us about hypothermia. With the decrease in body temperature, down went the heart rate and breathing until they became barely noticeable; the body burned its food so slowly that some Arctic animals could hibernate for six months of the year; the blood vessels shrank and the blood thickened. Research workers began to turn their minds to experiments on these hibernating animals to see how they might fare if they suddenly had to cope with artificial low temperatures. Would it injure their bodies—or their brains? For the question which still raised serious doubts in the minds of the surgeons was this: What would happen to the human brain if we subjected it to these low temperatures?

Another piece of the hypothermia jigsaw came from Holland, where a team of Dutch surgeons had started experiments at the same time as Bigelow. In Amsterdam, Professor Ite Boerema, a far-sighted doctor who has contributed much to surgery, believed like the Canadians that cooling might give him an open field in which to perform heart operations.

Boerema noted that shocks brought down the blood pressure, but did not damage a patient's brain; but he saw, too, that when deep anaesthesia stopped a patient's breathing the brain suffered damage, even though the heart continued to beat. Oxygen deprivation did the damage, and within minutes.

The Dutch professor had followed the trend towards the heart-lung machine which would keep the brain alive by circulating oxygenated blood. But, as he remarked, the problem his team set itself was not, "How do we supply the most sensitive tissues with sufficient oxygen during the exclusion of the heart?" Rather, it was, "How can we reduce as much as possible the quantity of oxygen required by the brain and elsewhere during a certain period?"

Boerema hit upon hypothermia as his method. But not for him the surface-cooling which Bigelow had employed with dogs; it meant that different parts of the body would cool unequally, and this would create the danger of shock on rewarming. The Dutchman's ingenious solution became a great contribution to the surgical onslaught on hypothermia. It was this: Use blood, the fluid which feeds every part of the body, as your cooling medium.

Two ways of cooling the blood stream struck the Dutchman —firstly, exposing the veins, chilling them and allowing the cooled blood to do the rest. Boerema chose to use the second method and bring the blood out of the body in tubes, run it through a refrigerator then return it into the blood stream.

Like Bigelow, he used animals which were first anaesthetized. The surgeon then opened a thigh artery and the neighbouring vein to slip the nozzle of his tubes into them. From the veins, blood flowed into a glass vessel which was immersed in an ice-bath. During the cooling the animals were given pure oxygen.

The Dutch team discovered that much depended on the rate

at which they cooled the animals. Too slow, and they proved difficult to revive; too quick and the heart began to flutter and falter. But they managed to bring the temperature down to 65 F.—several degrees lower than Bigelow—and keep it there for twenty minutes without experiencing difficulty reviving their experimental subjects.

At the end of their series of experiments, Boerema and his three colleagues had established that the heart could be cut out of the circulation for anything up to twenty minutes without brain damage. "It is possible," they commented, "that this method may eliminate the necessity for an artificial heart in cardiac surgery."

The next link in the hypothermia story came from a French surgeon, Henry Laborit, who was experimenting with various drugs to see if they exercised a lytic or calming effect on the body during illness or shock. Starting with local anaesthetics, he discovered that some of these blocked the nerves which control some internal organs independently of will power. Laborit, then working in Bizerta, went on to seek other drugs which might act as "general anaesthetics without anaesthesia". In other words, artificial hibernation.

The French discovery in the early fifties of chlorpromazine helped him to solve the problem. This powerful depressant, now widely used in mental hospitals as a tranquillizer, blocked the nerves, slowed the heart rate, the breathing and the body processes. Chlorpromazine had one other action which intrigued Laborit: it tugged down the patient's temperature by anything up to five or six degrees. Laborit combined this mind drug with other nerve-blocking agents in what he termed a Lytic Cocktail and used them to treat emergency cases in the Paris hospital to which he had moved.

From the practice of using the Lytic Cocktail to treat life-or-death cases it was only a step to hypothermia. Laborit set up a cooling room where the drug was dripped into the arm of patients who lay on a special trolley over which cool air could be blown. The French surgeon and his colleagues noticed that their drugs combated the shivering fits which worried surgeons in the operating theatre. Their patients went into a form of artificial hibernation, slowly and smoothly. The Laborit technique became standard practice in the Indo-China war, and French battle casualties had the drug-and-ice-water treatment to tide them over crises and reduce the shock of severe wounds. Service doctors reported from Indo-China that the Lytic Cocktail had cut their fatal casualties by about one in three.

Surgeons using hypothermia adopted the French technique when they were dealing with life-or-death cases and had to arrest bleeding. Brain surgeons have saved hundreds of lives with Laborit's drugs and cooling in the treatment of cerebral haemorrhage. Burns and other injuries have also yielded to this type of cold sleep.

Surgeons, however, still held grave doubts about relying solely on hypothermia during heart operations. It was a buxom young negro woman who, quite accidentally, helped to relieve their misgivings about the dangers of the new procedure.

She was 23, from the poor quarter of Chicago. For nine hours, from midday on the 8th of February, 1951, she had been drinking continuously. Unsteadily, she walked out into the cold, biting wind—it was 11 degrees below freezing point in the Middle West city—presumably to go home. But, in the dark she slipped on the icy pavement, tried to get to her feet but finally lost consciousness.

Eleven hours passed before a morning police patrol found her unconscious, her three-quarter length coat lying open over a thin dress. Her gloveless hands had stiffened, her feet, in light shoes, were swollen and her eyes looked glazed and dead. The policemen saw that she was not breathing, thought her beyond first-aid and drove her to the Michael Reese Hospital. But two doctors who looked harder at the small, stocky negress detected slow, irregular breathing. Her pulse, heard faintly over the heart, varied between 12 and 20 beats a minute—with long pauses in which the heart appeared to stop.

The intern and resident surgeon opened a vein in the crook of the left arm and injected a stimulant drug. They began blood transfusions and gave her oxygen through a mask until senior surgeon Dr. Harold Laufman arrived an hour later. Meticulously, Dr. Laufman examined the woman whose heart and breathing had picked up slightly, though the pulse still faltered.

She seemed completely frozen. He could not move the head from one side to the other; the unblinking eyes showed no reaction to strong light, and when the physician pressed on the lids the eyes beneath them felt, as he said, like glass. The woman's mouth had closed tightly and attempts to force it open failed. The arms and legs had stiffened and hardened and their pulse could neither be felt nor heard with a stethoscope. The only warmth the doctor could sense appeared to be in the lower abdomen.

He took the woman's temperature ninety minutes after she had been brought in. It was 64.4 degrees—34 degrees below normal, and when he went to take blood samples from an arm vein, the blood had thickened to such an extent that he could not draw it into the syringe.

By all the medical evidence, the woman ought to have died on the street. The Germans had recorded the same sort of case— the drunk who falls asleep and comes into hospital suffering from severe exposure. They had shown that 75 degrees seemed to be the critical temperature; no one had survived freezing below this level.

She should have died—and nearly did. Just before midday Dr. Laufman had to open her windpipe and pass an oxygen tube into it to permit the woman to breathe. It was only then that the staff at the Michael Reese believed the negress had a chance of pulling through.

The staff fixed the room temperature at 68 degrees—the temperature of the woman's body. They bandaged her arms and legs, then sat back to watch her condition. In the late afternoon her heart picked up its normal rhythm, though it frequently missed a beat; the temperature had now reached 80 degrees. But, more important, the eyes which had been glazed could now follow light and movement. By nightfall she began to speak, asking for her father whom she recognized when he came into the room.

Seventeen hours after her admission the doctors recorded that her temperature had become normal; her heart was beating fairly rapidly; the blood pressure was also within the usual limits. She could remember nothing about the twelve hours which preceded her collapse, but otherwise her mind seemed unaffected. Over the next two days, the woman regained her memory for the events just before she collapsed in the street. It looked like complete recovery, but a month after she had come into the hospital severe frostbite injuries forced the doctors to amputate parts of her lower legs and the fingers of the hands.

Laufman deduced from calculations that when the woman was found her temperature must have dropped to 60.8 degrees F. "To our knowledge," he said, "recovery from such low temperatures has not been recorded in man."

What had saved her? The surgeon said that alcohol, itself an anaesthetic, probably acted like light anaesthesia and offset the panic and the body disturbances which abrupt chilling cause. Drink does two other things which might have contributed to the woman's survival: it draws off heat from the deep tissues and dilates the surface blood vessels, creating a more rapid temperature drop; it might have kept the patient nourished by filtering through the stomach during the period of exposure and the early treatment.

Published in the *Journal of the American Medical Association,*

Laufman's report provoked more surgical interest in cooling as a form of anaesthesia for surgery. If a drunk woman could survive accidental freezing there appeared no good reason to suppose that scientific hypothermia would not work.

In Canada, research scientists followed the leads given by Bigelow; in America, Britain and elsewhere, doctors and surgeons eagerly tackled the problems of frozen-sleep for patients.

Perhaps the most dramatic work was going on at this time behind the Iron Curtain, in a laboratory in Belgrade. There, a tall, good-looking Serbian had decided to test the effects of extreme cold on rats. Radoslav Andjus was young enough not to know the current medical dogma on rats: they could not, said all the pundits, be revived after freezing below 55 degrees Fahrenheit. Andjus ought to have appreciated this and abandoned any thoughts of repeating previous experiments. But at that time no Belgrade University library existed; it had been bombed and gutted by fire. So Dr. Andjus began to chill rats to progressively lower temperatures, and, without knowing it, established new records for reviving them from below 55 degrees.

The Slav scientist came to Paris for a year to continue his animal experiments. At that time in the same research centre was a young American who had previously worked at Britain's National Institute for Medical Research in Mill Hill. Seeing Andjus's experiments reminded the American that Dr. Alan Parkes and Dr. Audrey Smith had done similar studies with cells and tissues. When he returned to London he mentioned the young Belgrade doctor who was obtaining such wonderful results with rats. So, a few months later, the lean, dark-haired figure found himself walking through the entrance to the tall building on the outskirts of London to demonstrate how he froze rats to the point where they showed no signs of life and then revived them. Dr. Audrey Smith and Professor Otto

Edholm watched, were impressed and then invited the young Yugoslav to come and work at the institute for a year to take the experiments further.

The two British Government scientists watched Andjus place the animals in jars packed in ice so that they inhaled their own spent breath until they became drowsy and lightly anaesthetized by the cold. Then he dowsed them in iced water until their body temperatures had fallen to between freezing point and two degrees above it. Their breathing and hearts at this stage reached a standstill and he left them like this for a full hour. Then Andjus warmed the frozen animals by placing a hot metal element to their chests and puffing air into their lungs through a rubber mask. When he arrived at Mill Hill he reported that one out of five of the rats recovered. For animals which did not hibernate it was an impressive score, and changed the current thinking about life at low temperature.

But the Mill Hill laboratories thought they could improve on Andjus's work. They asked him to apply for a year's leave of absence from Belgrade and join their staff. Within a year, Andjus and his collaborator, Dr. Smith, had devised a method of reviving at least three-quarters of the animals. This they did by warming the heart by high-frequency radio waves. Later, Audrey Smith found that ordinary electric light bulbs placed round the animals guaranteed an even better percentage of survivors—though they still had to breathe into the lungs.

Word got round about the strange experiment at Mill Hill, and when Andjus and Audrey Smith were invited to demonstrate their research to a meeting of the Physiological Society, the small room in the London Institute could not hold the eminent scientists who turned up to watch the freezing and revival of rats.

But what was happening to the animals during these periods of freezing? Dr. Alan Parkes suggested to the team that they should let the psychologists at University College, London, put them through intelligence tests before and after they had recovered from cold storage. The rats astonished the psychologists. The animals first did a simple I.Q. test such as finding their food at the end of a maze. After their freezing ordeal they galloped through the same routine without showing signs of losing their skill.

One other important factor emerged. The complete mental black-out which occurred seemed to have no effect on the brain cells or the intelligence of the animals. A series of tests made on the rats showed that the signals from their brains made no trace on the electrical recording machine when the body temperature fell below 64 degrees Fahrenheit. And yet the rats went through their food and swimming puzzles, as easily after as before freezing.

The brain physiologists had to reorientate their thinking after these experiments. They had held that when the brain ceased to emit signals, all memory of preceding events would be washed out. Here, however, were rats whose brains had lain silent for an hour or more in frozen sleep; to all intents they were dead. And yet their memories had come through this trial unimpaired. Of course, they were rats—they had a very primitive brain—we should have to see what happens to the more sensitive human brain, said the physiologists.

If the rat proved versatile, its second cousin, the hamster, outdid it in laboratory tricks. These golden-brown household pets who are natural hibernators showed, without any doubt, that they could be put into a state of suspended animation and then resuscitated after several hours.

Dr. Audrey Smith describes these animals when they were frozen down to 41 degrees below zero as having board-stiff bodies. She was able to hold them quite straight and stiff by putting two fingers under their thin tails and pointed snouts. Half of their body water had converted to ice in the freezing process. Nonetheless, they revived with their full faculties.

From lumps of cold, seemingly inanimate matter, the hamsters came round when the temperature rose to 50 degrees. Their hearts and breathing, which had stopped, picked up, and bouts of shivering helped the rewarming operation.

In 1953, the Medical Research Council, Britain's panel of leading doctors and scientists, began to take an active interest in the hypothermia experiments at Mill Hill, their biggest laboratories. At that time the Council was trying to make up its mind whether the deep-freeze principles might be applied to surgery or medical treatment.

The laboratory laid on a private viewing for the eminent men, and they wandered round looking at the frozen animals—and incidentally uncovering a fact which had escaped the research workers. One of the Council members became so interested in these rock-hard animals that he picked one up and tried to bend its brittle ears. When they thawed out the hamster, Dr. Smith saw that its ears had suffered frostbite from the rough handling while it was frozen.

The hamster experiments raised several important and intriguing puzzles in the minds of the medical experts. These animals obviously had been frozen into a state of suspended animation, had spent a whole hour in some limbo between life and death. Had anyone ignorant of the experiments been asked if they were dead, he would not have hesitated to say, "Yes."

What was death? Clearly, the work on rats and hamsters indicated there were two kinds of death—clinical and biological. It seemed to many research workers in Britain when they studied the Mill Hill results that the rule-of-thumb methods of diagnosing clinical death might have to be revised. What of the many who were picked up out of the sea and in the mountains during the war? they asked. Many of those might have been alive when they were pronounced dead. It was a disturbing question, but fortunately no-one would ever be able to answer it.

13

Frozen-Sleep Surgery

TO SURGEONS and research workers it became apparent that they would solve the mystery of what happened to frozen human beings in one place only: the operating table. By 1952, a fat dossier of experimental evidence had accumulated on animals and the odd accidental case of hypothermia. Someone had to venture to do surgery to see whether cooling made an effective anaesthetic and if it would protect the body and brain during operations where the heart was excluded.

Again, the team at Minneapolis blazed the trail. Over the border, in Toronto, they had worked with dogs, so two surgeons at the Minnesota Medical School began duplicating Bigelow's ice-blanket technique with animals and arrived at his conclusions. Dr. F. John Lewis and his colleague, Dr. Mansur Taufic, decided to test the statement about cardiac surgery in the Canadian report. First they put the idea to Richard L. Varco, one of the team which later pioneered cross-circulation and the heart-lung machine. Varco approved; moreover, he found their first patient.

She lay in the University hospital, a five-year-old girl who weighed less than 30 lbs. Frail and sickly, she had come into the cardiac department with a loud, blowing murmur and exhaustion. The doctors who passed a tube into an upper chamber of the heart found the tell-tale mixing of spent and fresh blood which meant that a tear had appeared in the dividing wall of the auricles.

With the support of Varco, the girl became the first patient to undergo frozen-sleep surgery. On the 2nd of September, 1952, they prepared the machine which would force frozen spirit through rubber blankets and a warm bath to revive the girl after the operation. They needed nothing else.

The girl was first put to sleep with pentothal, then, to relax the muscles and prevent shivering which might exhaust her and raise the blood pressure, they injected curare, the poison with which South American Indians tip their arrows. As this collapsed the lungs, the anaesthetist kept her breathing by squeezing oxygen into them through a rubber bag.

They used light hypothermia, resolving to bring down the temperature to 80° F. —just over 18 below the normal body heat. Their experimental studies had indicated that this temperature would allow them to clamp off the heart for about ten minutes while they operated. Beyond this critical time the brain might demand oxygen which was not there, and its sensitive cells might die.

Ninety minutes it took for the frozen fluid in the blankets to cause the temperature to drop to the level which the surgeons wanted. They then opened the chest and tied off the blood vessels leading in and out of the heart. There were no signs of shock; the heart beat had certainly slowed, but still remained steady.

The right upper chamber was opened, and there in the centre of the heart lay a hole just under an inch in diameter. While one of their staff called out the minutes as they passed the surgeons raced against the clock to run the tear together with silk stitches. In five and a half minutes they placed the last suture and unclamped the heart to allow blood to flow freely to it and to the brain.

The operation took two minutes under an hour. The girl's temperature at that point measured 79 F., with still no signs of the heart flutter which hypothermia can induce.

Rewarming merely meant putting the girl into a bath of warm water and watching her temperature as it began to climb. In 35 minutes the thermometer read 96.8, and they wheeled her out of the operating theatre to recover from the anaesthetic. She was up in a day; the doctors noticed the murmur had gone; and on the eleventh day after the operation, the girl went home to lead a normal life.

Hypothermia had ceased to be only a series of research projects; it had been written into the surgical text-books, and had proved itself to be a useful adjunct to the surgeon in heart operations. Several surgeons immediately followed the example of the Minneapolis group and began to introduce hypothermia as a routine in their operating theatres.

Notable among these was Dr. Henry Swan, of the University of Colorado School of Medicine in Denver. Swan discarded the blanket method of cooling and brought an ordinary bath into the operating theatre. Lightly anaesthetized, the patients were then placed in a bath of ice water, their hands taped to the side to prevent the fingers from cooling too much. To stop shivering fits, the Denver surgeon gave curare, the muscle relaxant.

Swan adopted a method of rewarming his patients which Bigelow had advocated and used experimentally. He wrapped them in a dry blanket round which he passed coils attached to a short-wave generator. By passing short-wave current through the coils the patients were warmed in depth. This deep-ray technique seemed an advance on the warm-bath method which Lewis had employed.

A hundred cases of heart disease were treated with this ice-bath technique. Of these, fifty-nine had defects which called for open-heart surgery. Swan reported fourteen deaths which could be attributed to hypothermia; he said, too, that some of his patients suffered from violent heart flutter during the cooling and rewarming; but he pronounced that the method, in his opinion, was "highly effective and quite safe".

Both Lewis and Swan came to the American Surgical Association congress in Philadelphia, in April, 1955, to report fully on their cold-sleep operations. Swan, a blunt and descriptive talker, criticized the "blind surgery" which most people were then practising and said no one could hope, by groping with the fingers, to accomplish as much as the surgeon using open-heart techniques.

Swan put it this way: "Finger vision is capable of limited success, and bears the same relation to real vision in surgery that it does in life—one can read Braille with moderate facility, but the chromatic values of the Mona Lisa escape one, and to shoot a winging mallard or to fly an airplane is impossible.

"That the blind but educated finger is capable of accomplishing much within the heart is to be fully admitted, and much admired; that it should be considered as the best method in the long run is absurd." Swan pleaded that the element of risk should decide the method to be used; his figures proved that hypothermia was worthwhile.

The attack on blind surgery brought angry or equally sarcastic comments from several surgeons who had done hundreds of valve repairs with only their fingers and skill to guide them. They threw back at Swan the fact that many of them had never seen heart flutter during their operations; and that the mortality in hypothermic procedure was too high. The high death-rate did, in fact, cause many surgeons in America, Britain and the Continent to think twice about cooling their patients in anything but emergency treatment.

Some of the doubts about hypothermia were crystallized by Dr. Charles Bailey, the surgeon who had revived the Souttar operation for mitral stenosis. After a series of experiments, Bailey had tried hypothermia on a patient a few days before the successful operation by Lewis and Taufic, but the patient had died. He pushed on, taking very poor-risk patients with serious heart defects; though he had to report that thirteen out of twenty died. The death-rate, he considered, was running too high and said so at a conference attended by Bigelow, Lewis and Swan.

It was the old story about new medical technique. The surgeon had to accept patients rejected by orthodox standards and jeopardize his reputation by trying to save them with methods which were fraught with difficulties and unknowns. But hypothermia had attracted several brilliant operators, and they decided, despite the hostile attitude of many of their contemporaries, to carry on.

No one made light of the problems. The heart spasm seen too often in hypothermia remained perhaps the biggest. When temperatures dropped below 86 F., surgeons noted all too often that the heart was wriggling ineffectually and the electro-cardiogram recording a ragged, sinister scribble. It could be reversed, this fibrillation, by applying a small voltage to the heart; but in many cases the rhythm never steadied, the heart became useless as a pump and squirmed to a halt. Drugs helped, but did not stop the condition.

The time limit imposed by hypothermia raised snags. Isolation of the heart for eight or ten minutes gave surgeons too little time to enter the heart and sew up complicated defects. Rewarming patients after cooling brought about changes in the blood acid, bleeding in some cases, and death. To correct the blood acidity some hospitals used the simple remedy for indigestion—bicarbonate of soda.

But the pioneers of hypothermia had to meet another challenge. The heart-lung machine had taken shape and was already installed in the operating theatres of the Mayo Clinic and in Minneapolis. In Sweden and Britain these machines had come through their experimental period and surgeons were now working on their first human cases. Would cooling have any place in heart surgery when the machines began to beat the problems which faced those who favoured pure hypothermia?

The brave ones carried on. But the arrival of the machines split the hypothermia field into two: those who intended to use the machine while they cooled their patients, and the others who sought means of cooling without an artificial heart and lungs.

Some of the most emphatic misgivings came from the man who had done so much pioneering work at the Wilhelmina Gasthuis Surgical Clinic in Amsterdam. Professor Ite Boerema threw the weight of seven years' study and experimental work behind his arguments that hypothermia, and even heart-lung machines, could damage not only the brain but the heart itself. Machines, he said mean diluting the blood and making running repairs which might themselves give trouble once the heart has been keyed back into the circulation.

Hypothermia seemed better than machines. But surgeons still had to overcome the obstacles. Blood cooling entailed using anti-clotting substances which could cause death; surface cooling, on the other hand, gave different temperature readings all over the body which added to the risks; the oxygen depletion might leave some organs damaged; and, finally, the method left the surgeon watching the clock as well as his patient.

Boerema proposed a characteristically clever and daring solution: couple cooling with oxygen saturation and perform the surgery inside a sealed, high-pressure chamber. The Royal Dutch Navy willingly lent the stocky, bespectacled professor a diving bell, and he began his experiments with animals.

Boerema, the first man to suggest bloodstream cooling in hypothermia, abandoned this technique in favour of ice-pack treatment which did not involve doctoring the patient's blood. Temperatures below 79 F. he considered introduced dangerous heart flutter, so he determined to cool to a minimum of 80 F. The Dutch surgeon designed an operating cabinet, a large wooden box with a slatted, open top through which hot air could be blown. The patient lay on a net over the box.

The patient was slowly cooled with ice packs and the operation performed. To prevent temperature drop during the surgery, controlled streams of hot air were blown through the box. But Boerema did not follow the procedure of other surgeons when he had finished the heart repair. He kept the chest open, placed a transparent blood hood over the hot box and rewarmed the patient this way. It took an hour and meant conducting the operation in two stages; but the surgeon contended that this method ruled out the danger of closing the wound without being aware of bleeding from it; also, it made for uniform rewarming.

The system worked in several operations on children. However, the surgeon pointed out that this form of moderate hypothermia gave twelve minutes at the most to operate inside the heart. It was not enough, so he looked around for means to extend this period.

Here, he brought in the pressure tank. The twelve-minute limit had been fixed because then the dearth of oxygen in the brain made the business too hazardous. What, asked Boerema, if we could increase the oxygen supply to the brain by taking the operating theatre inside the pressure tank? With the help of technicians from the Dutch Navy, he designed the pressure vessel to accommodate himself, his staff and a patient.

Boerema argued thus: Lower the body temperature to a safe level of 80 F. and you cut the oxygen demand of the tissues by half. If you then put the patient into a chamber and pump in three times the normal atmospheric pressure, the tissues could be charged with about six times their normal quota of oxygen. You would then have created an oxygen store in the body which would permit the surgeon to stop the circulation long enough to do intricate heart operations.

So, for the first time in surgical history, a whole theatre moved into a form of naval diving bell. Some of his staff became light-headed working at this pressure—"a slight impairment of intellectual functions," in Boerema's words—but they had to get used to it while they experimented with animals. They had little room to move; they sat round the operating table; and when they emerged it meant the decompression drill which divers undergo to prevent nitrogen bubbles filtering into their blood stream and causing "the bends".

However, Boerema's theory was right. The tissues did soak up the pure oxygen which the experimental subjects were given. The Dutchman was able to show that the twelve-minute period could be extended to forty-five minutes using high-pressure techniques—without damage to the brain. Oxygen seemed to protect the heart as well, for the Dutch surgeons found it recovered more easily from the fluttering which hypothermia often provoked.

In July, 1956, Boerema announced the work of his team to the European Cardiovascular Surgery Society, and said in his summing up: "That it is quite possible to carry out surgical procedures in a high-pressure tank which is equipped as an operating theatre, is proven. Both surgeons and anaesthetists are able to work well under these conditions. The tissues, saturated with oxygen and inactive are probably able to endure a long period of circulatory arrest, which, under other circumstances would entail a danger far too great for the individual."

The Dutch team operated successfully on many cases using hypothermia. Their high-pressure surgery also made it possible to shut down the circulation long enough to do cardiac operations. As a by-product of the research the Dutch surgeons found they could cure two other dangerous conditions: gas gangrene and coal gas poisoning. Gas gangrene, caused by a microbe which thrives in the absence of oxygen, normally meant amputation of the affected limb. By putting these cases into the high-pressure chamber and saturating their tissues with oxygen, Boerema and his colleagues killed off the gangrene germs and removed the need for amputation.

Coal gas could at one time be treated only by transfusion because the gas has a fatal affinity for haemoglobin, the red constituent of the blood which transports oxygen to the cells. Coal gas sticks to this fraction of the blood 300 times more readily than oxygen. But feeding poisoned patients oxygen at three times normal pressure forced it into the tissues and saved lives. This method was also pioneered by a team of doctors at Glasgow University.

With his pressure chamber, Boerema conceived an even more revolutionary idea—life without blood at all. Apart from acting as a form of waterway for food supplies to the cells or to carry chemical agents, blood mainly effects the exchange of oxygen and carbon dioxide in the tissues. Boerema set about establishing the fact that his pressurized oxygen could supply these tissues with very dilute blood. When he had proof he posed himself the question: Why not use just a chemical fluid? Animal experiments in his chamber showed that a clear, watery solution of saline with sugars as nutrients would amply support life. His results convinced him that surgery could be performed by draining the body of its blood and replacing it with this clear, limpid fluid. Not only could the surgeon suspend the circulation for long periods; he would also have a completely clear view of the repair he was carrying out, and no blood to worry him. Boerema has not yet graduated to using this technique in routine operations, but feels it has immense possibilities.

14

Switching Life Off—and On

A s t h e first flush of enthusiasm about hypothermia faded, even the most sanguine among surgeons realized in the mid-fifties that they needed much more basic research before they could open the way to the heart. A certain academic quibbling went on about whether to use body or blood cooling; whether to bring in the heart-lung machine just in case; whether the 86-degree line or the 10-minute limit would ever be passed without heart arrest. While some surgeons marked time, others diligently backtracked through the literature. A clever piece of research by Dr. Frank Gollan and a group of doctors in America convinced many of the doubters that hypothermia did have a future.

Gollan, a man with an encyclopaedic knowledge of hypothermia, decided to see how long animals would survive cooling if their circulation were kept going with a heart-lung machine. He pushed the leads of the heart-lung apparatus through the large artery and vein in the leg until they sat close to the heart. The lungs he ventilated with a mechanical respirator while he pumped blood through a stainless-steel cooling coil immersed in ice water.

Then Gollan and his two associates from Vanderbilt University medical school, Nashville, Tennessee, cooled the animals down to as low as 75 degrees. They were able to clamp off the heart for as much as an hour with very little blood flow through their machine. The animals were rewarmed by replacing the freezing liquid round the coil with hot water.

Gollan's experiments established one thing: with the pump to keep circulation flowing the heart did not go into fibrillation; nor did the brain suffer. It seemed that by keeping the heart supplied with fresh blood the big barrier to hypothermia might be breached.

In Britain, several surgeons had followed up the work done at Mill Hill on hibernating animals. One of the first men to appreciate the significance of cooling in cardiac surgery was Sir Russell Brock, who set up a unit at Guy's Hospital to study experimentally the effects of hypothermia.

In February, 1955, he and his assistant, Mr. Donald Ross, reported that they had operated on twenty patients using a new method of blood-stream cooling. They started first with the system Boerema had evolved—draining the blood from a vein and pushing it back through an artery. But, though this worked well in the laboratory, it failed in the operating theatre; the blood flow fell as the heart slowed and the cannulation of an artery created the risk of a blood clot after the operation.

The two Guy's surgeons decided to try a new method of cooling only the blood flowing through the veins. Some form of pressure was needed, so they devised a hand pump which pushed the venous flow through a cooling coil round the body. To get to the great veins draining the blood into the heart they pushed their pump leads through veins in the neck and the thigh, but this again raised snags.

Ross then hit on the idea of tying the leads of the pump directly into the mouth of these veins through the upper right chamber of the heart. It meant opening the heart before cooling could start, though this had the advantages of giving the surgeons time to look at the heart and diagnose the defects. Ross's idea worked, and as the surgeons said in their report, "This we consider is a great practical step forward in the clinical use of hypothermia."

The new technique allowed the surgeons to cool and rewarm

patients quickly by altering the temperature of the fluid surrounding the coil outside the body. But it did nothing to offset
the main objections to hypothermia—heart failure and the time
limit on operations. Brock and Ross devised a method of
feeding oxygen-rich blood to the heart during such operations
to prevent heart flutter, but this made no general appeal to
their colleagues.

Hypothermia lost many of its adherents in those years of
doubt. Many surgeons, discouraged by the way in which the
heart reacted to cold, turned instead to the machines which
had proved safe in long operations. But the surgeons with
heart-lung machines had struck snags, too. The technique of
stopping the heart with potassium injection sometimes caused
the heart to behave erratically and was thought to impair the
function of its main muscles.

Not all had given up hope of using hypothermia in heart
operations. Lillehei and his group at Minneapolis were trying a
new technique which would combine the heart-lung machine
with cooling of the heart alone. They tapped warm blood from
the machine and passed it through a bath of ice and into the
heart with a small tube. By October, 1958, they had started
applying the method in the operating theatre. At 20 degrees F.
they discovered that the heart came to a complete standstill and
could be held there for as long as open-heart surgery lasted.
They were relieved to see that no heart fluttering developed as
they warmed the organ.

A cold heart meant that less oxygen was required to keep it
alive, and this gave the surgeon certain advantages over the
chemical technique of stopping the organ. From the moment
the Minnesota University group published their results, hypothermia took on a new impetus as an ally of the machine.

Among those experimenting with the cooling method were
three surgeons at the Naval Hospital in Bethesda, Maryland.
Throughout 1958 they had tried local cooling of animal

hearts and convinced themselves that it would work with patients.

In the spring came their patient—a U.S. Navy yeoman, thirty-three years old, well-built and athletic. A few months before he had developed pains in his chest and breathlessness when he ran and his unit doctor had diagnosed heart trouble.

At the Naval Hospital they went through the routine X-rays, catheterization and tracings of the heart. These all pointed to the same thing: a weak and strained left heart chamber and the possibility of a recent coronary attack. Even with the stethoscope, the surgeons could hear a blowing murmur over the left heart and the muffled sound of the main valve at the mouth of the left ventricle.

The surgeons, Dr. Harold C. Urschel, Charles A. Hufnagel and Lt. Jack J. Greenberg, realized they faced a defect in the aortic valve through which blood is pumped to the main artery. They had used a novel idea to cool the hearts of animals. Could they test their technique on this case?

Their equipment consisted of a heart-lung machine fitted with a cooling and heating unit in its blood circuit. Two flasks of ice-cold solution would serve to cool the heart to a standstill.

On the 20th of May, 1959, they exposed the heart by splitting the breastbone and connected the leads from the heart-lung machine to the main blood vessels. Slowly they cooled the body to 85 F., the point at which the heart might begin to falter. Then, keeping the machine going, Urschel split the artery and probed through the nick with a gloved finger to the three-leaved valve. There, an inch below the valve, lay a tough ring of tissue which was choking the outflow of blood from the heart.

To cut the tissue away would involve stopping the heart, so the surgeons decided to put the new technique into practice.

Into the nick in the main blood vessel one of them placed the thin tube which led from an ice flask. Round the tube he pulled stitches to keep it in place while he allowed the ice-cold fluid to drain into the arteries which fed the heart itself. Another surgeon swabbed the four chambers with the same icy liquid—and gradually the heart flagged, halted and, in thirty seconds, collapsed limply. The chilled heart was emptied of blood and the surgeon got to work opening the aorta and excising the fibrous tissue which blocked this main channel. For twenty minutes the heart lay, cold and inert, until he had finished. To warm and restart the heart, the surgeons merely loosened the clamps from the blood vessels around it and let blood at normal temperature flow into its arteries.

The Bethesda groups did several other operations to confirm the validity of the method before publishing their results. Their work quashed many misgivings about chilling the heart, and from 1959 hypothermia began to take over in cardiac surgery.

Charles Hufnagel evolved another way of applying local cooling—by immersing the heart in ice crystals to stop its action. The heart-lung machine still kept body circulation moving while the heart was excluded. Then freezing crystals were placed around the heart while the surgeon operated. In several British hospitals the "frozen-heart" method has been done dozens of times with great success. The crystals are made by standing bottles of salt water in crushed ice until the salt solution begins to crystallize. With these crystals, the heart can be stopped in a minute and restarted easily.

One of the first hospitals to put the Hufnagel method to use was Bigelow's unit at Toronto. There they developed a machine which would short-circuit the heart and lungs while cooling the patient slightly. To stop the heart they surrounded it with ice-crystals.

At the beginning of 1961 they operated on 15-year-old Arthur Perry, from Uxbridge, Ontario—and cooled his heart with ice to only three degrees above freezing point. Other surgeons had been content with something six or seven times greater. The surgeons repaired a defective aortic valve while the heart was frozen and still. The boy was kept at just under normal temperature—and during the later stages of the operation even lay with his eyes open talking to the surgeons.

Still another technique makes use of the heart-lung machine to arrest the heart. The blood goes through a heat-exchanger in the machine which slowly cools it and passes it back into the body. Since the circulation is moving and supplying the heart with oxygen, the dreaded fibrillation is avoided and the heart and body can be cooled to very low temperatures.

By protecting the heart against arrest the machines had taken care of one big obstacle during cold surgery. But one other big barrier in hypothermia still existed—the time limitation for complete circulatory arrest. Many of its adherents had given up hope of ever practising deep cooling by itself in heart surgery. One who had not was Charles Drew, a surgeon at the Westminster Hospital in London.

Drew had followed heart research throughout the world for more than ten years, picking up experience and information in visits to America and elsewhere and quietly trying out several methods in his laboratory. For some time he worked with the Lillehei machine, using this for stopped-heart surgery.

But hypothermia attracted him. And several features of the research and experience with cooling convinced him that surgeons could take the body well below 86 degrees without endangering life. Andjus and Smith had done it with rats which did not hibernate; Gollan had proved with his animals that the heart might be cooled and arrested for an hour or more providing there was a low blood flow; and then one could point to the case of the woman who had survived after her body had dropped to a temperature of no more than 48 degrees.

The woman, with widespread cancer, came into the University of Minnesota hospital in Minneapolis for treatment by

F. John Lewis, the man who performed the first successful hypothermia operation. Lewis and a colleague, Dr. S. A. Niazi, cooled the woman to 50 degrees below normal temperature with ice blankets. Her heart, brain and lungs came to a standstill for forty-five minutes—but she recovered with no signs of damage to any part of the body or her brain.

Drew and two of his colleagues favoured not surface refrigeration but the more efficient method of cooling the blood stream through a heat-exchanger circuit.

With the pump which Lillehei had adopted for his heart-lung machine, they tried experimentally to take blood from the left side of the heart, cool it and push it back into the arteries. But with only one pump they found the blood failed to circulate properly through the lungs; the heart, too, failed time and again.

Since this heart failure seemed to run hand in hand with hypothermia below 85 degrees F., Drew began to reason that he needed not one pump, but two. With a dual pump he could take over the function of both the main chambers of the heart and keep the circulation moving until the cooling process halted the heart.

Their first double-pump was crude. They had trouble with the heat exchanger, a 100-foot coil of plastic tube which was cooled with a mixture of alcohol and dry ice. But the apparatus worked.

The principle had the simplicity of genius. Blood would be drawn from the receiving chamber of the left heart, forced through the heat exchanger and then returned cold to an artery in the thigh. One pump did this.

While the cooling took place the other pump was tied into the circuit—one end into the right receiving chamber and the other into the outflow valve. As cooling progressed, this pump kept circulating blood round the lungs. Drew had thus dispensed with the most complicated and troublesome half of the heart-lung machine—the mechanical lung.

They started experiments with animals which were taken down in temperature to 40 degrees F. and then rewarmed. In two cases the heart and circulation were stopped for thirty minutes. All but two of the animals died, though in some instances this resulted from inexperience, the surgeons confessed. The Westminster team were disappointed with the experiments—but looked on the two survivors as proof that hypothermia could be induced quickly through bloodstream cooling without incurring a penalty in either the brain or the body. The fault, they thought, lay in the cooling circuit of the apparatus.

The surgeons scrapped the plastic tubing which had tended to impede the blood flow and substituted heat-exchange tubes which proved more efficient. The next series of tests supported their previous findings; the apparatus worked.

At the beginning of 1959, Drew, working with a child specialist, Dr. Ian Anderson, decided to take the new machine into the operating theatre. Their experiments had done nothing to answer one big question: would the machine and the novel technique work as well on crippled hearts as on healthy ones? They chose children with incurable heart defects.

With the first child they had bad luck—the sort of setback which had driven Gibbon to abandon surgery with the first heart-lung machine for a long period. When they opened the chest they found that the heart was beating very weakly and it proved difficult to tie the ends of the machine into both upper chambers. But they dropped the child's temperature to 59 degrees—much lower than it had ever been before in a human patient—and stopped the heart for forty-six minutes. Drew managed to repair one of the holes in the heart before he started rewarming. The surgeon noticed that the heart took up its normal beat without the dreaded fluttering. The operation ended; the child showed no signs of ill-effects. But nearly two hours later, the surgeon watching the regular scrawl of the electrocardiogram, suddenly observed it change character.

The sharp peaks which indicated the action of the heart's main pumping chambers took up a new, slow rhythm. The heart had gone into block; the upper and lower chambers were beating independently.

Quickly they incised his chest and the surgeon began to massage the heart. An electric pacemaker was used to try to re-establish the heart rhythm. But in vain. Only one comfort remained. The case amply confirmed the possibility of cooling to low temperatures, stopping the heart and rewarming quickly. The heart abnormalities seemed to present no obstacle to using the machine.

Drew went on to do two other children and both these operations bore out his theory and experiments.

For the first time a surgeon had stopped not only the heart, but the whole of the body. The clinical death which Audrey Smith had spoken of five years before had been realized in the operating theatre. For forty-five minutes or more the patient could be a cadaver, with his heart, breathing, his body and even his brain as still as death . . . and yet thirty minutes later wake up as though nothing had happened.

Drew had not yet finished. His technique had succeeded but his machine needed improvements. While he worked with the apparatus which three of his colleagues had helped to build he cast around for a more efficient system of cooling and heating blood.

The Westminster surgeon launched himself on a study of heat transfer and found this bristled with as many problems as heart surgery. At the Imperial College of Science, in London, a professor mentioned to him that a pupil of his, David Shore, could probably help. Drew located Shore at the new town of Crawley, working with a firm of engineers, called A.P.V. The designer knew nothing about medicine, but the two men got together and ran over the technical and medical problems.

Drew's wants were disarmingly simple—but gave Shore enough to keep him busy for the next two years. The mechanical heart should have two pumps which would replace the ventricles and adjust to run at almost any speed. This was easy: the De Bakey type of roller pump already existed. More tricky was the heat exchanger. "But," said Shore, "we had tackled this problem with many other liquids—even including cream. We had, however, to overcome the big problem of blood damage at temperatures between 32 degrees F. and 104 F. at which the machine would run. The exchanger had also to function with very low amounts of blood, anything from three-quarters of a pint. It took me nine months to satisfy myself and the surgeon with the answer. The long cylinder with four separate blood channels proved itself with long trials to be perfect for the job."

The cooling and warming unit, however, required a lot of intricate design. Safeguards had to be built in to prevent failure while the unit was working and the designer had to ensure that it would switch smoothly from cold to warm during any emergency in the operating theatre.

The finished machine did everything that Drew had demanded—and it solved many of the problems of cardiac surgery. With the heart-lung machine the oxygenator had always given more trouble than the rest of the apparatus. The patient whose lungs had been isolated from his circulation for an hour or more often woke up with "wet lungs" and a cough which made nursing difficult in the early stages. It was while Drew was using the heart-lung machine that he noticed the chest troubles and wondered if the patient's own lungs might be made to play their part during cardiac surgery. The A.P.V. machine ruled out lung trouble.

Unlike some heart-lung machines this one did not need large volumes of blood to prime it; it solved, too, another headache for the heart surgeon: where to get donors. With heart-lung machines the blood had to be fresh and this meant calling donors to hospitals on the day of the operations; this procedure virtually ruled out emergency heart operations. Drew's machine took blood which might be many days in store, and it did much less damage to it than the other machines. By October, 1960, the apparatus had come through its laboratory tests and the surgeon began to carry out experiments which demonstrated that it was good enough for the operating theatre. With this robot heart "cold surgery" took a tremendous leap forward—to the point where the surgeon could almost abolish the life force at will, and then recreate it. The cleverest hibernating animal could not switch off his heart, lungs and brain completely—but the surgeon had achieved just this.

In the ward of a large London teaching hospital the clock hands point to 9 a.m. and the slender, fair-haired boy watches a doctor and a nurse approach his bed. He knows that today he will have an operation on the heart which has caused him so much trouble since he was born; that a surgeon will sew up a hole and this will allow him to run and play games like other children. He is six years of age.

"This won't hurt," says the doctor as he swabs the boy's arm with cold spirit. The syringe contains some clear liquid and the boy feels nothing as this is injected slowly into his arm. In a few minutes he feels pleasantly drowsy, though his mouth is drier than he can remember. The pethidine and atropine which will help to kill the pain and keep his heart steady have begun to take effect. In an hour they will come for him with a trolley and wheel him into the operating theatre.

The operating theatre is a large room, its windows overlooking some of the high buildings of the city. The table lies under a powerful arc lamp and by its side the intricate plumbing of the anaesthetic apparatus. But the staff are assembling another, more curious machine. From sacks they take the components which have been sterilized in dry heat and fit them into position.

First come two plastic cylinders eleven inches long. These are placed on the machine with their plastic tubes leading into the two heavy pumps sitting in their square mountings on the machine trolley. Two more tubes sheeted in thin plastic will later be tied into the heart. Behind the large pressure gauge is a socket into which the theatre staff are fitting a long, polished drum which they have just put together. This heat-exchanger will cool and rewarm the blood before and after the operation. Its four cylinders fit closely together inside the stainless-steel outer jacket of the drum.

The cylinders are rifled like a gun barrel to send the blood spiralling evenly round them in four streams so that it cools and heats quickly. The rifling distributes the blood so well that the machine can cool or rewarm the patient in half an hour though primed with only one-and-a-half pints of blood.

Basically, the machine could hardly be more simple. Four plastic leads, three of which are tied into the heart and the other into an artery in the leg. The two plastic cylinders act as reservoirs for the blood from the upper chambers of the heart; the two pumps take over from the main pumping chambers and keep the circulation going; and a heater and refrigerator alter the blood temperature.

No artificial oxygenator is needed. The machine merely keeps the blood flowing until it has cooled to between 10 and 15 degrees Centigrade. At this low temperature the body can manage without oxygen for almost an hour, and perhaps more.

The last screws have been tightened and the pumps tested with saline solution to make sure the pressure is right. The surgical team, in their green gowns and white caps, stand by to wait for the patient. In the anaesthetic room, a doctor has opened a vein in the boy's arm and is injecting a straw-coloured liquid into it which sends him to sleep in several seconds. His body is painted with a yellow, antiseptic solution and he is ready for the operating theatre.

The pump, standing ready, will not be needed for the best part of an hour. But while the surgeons get busy, the pumps are primed with salt solution and tested to see that the cooling and the heating unit works properly.

The anaesthetist passes a breathing tube into the windpipe and feeds a mixture of nitrous oxide and ether through this to keep the patient lightly anaesthetized. Now, he slips a syringe into the socket of the needle which he left in the arm vein and injects a minute dose of curare which will relax the muscles and stop any shivering during the cooling period. A respirator pump keeps a steady flow of air going to the lungs.

The surgeon and his assistants turn to the task of fixing measuring devices all over the body. Temperature probes are placed at three points which will tell how the cooling and re-warming progress; leads are attached for the electrocardiogram and the electroencephalogram which will record the heart and the brain waves during the operation. A pen recorder with several channels starts monitoring this information and the surgeon looks at the ragged but rhythmic waves from the brain and the peaked writing from the heart as they come through.

An assistant sings out the temperature in Centigrade: 35.8 ... 35.9 ... 35.7 ...

The first incision is made—a small nick in the left groin baring the artery in which the surgeon will later place one of the stainless-steel ends of the pump leads. A similar cut in the right groin uncovers another artery which will be cannulated to give blood-pressure readings.

The apparatus is primed with one-and-a-half pints of blood to which heparin is added to prevent clotting. The surgeon and his staff are all at their posts, ready to begin the real work of the operation.

The deep, bold cut is made down the breast bone, which is split carefully so that the lungs are not pierced. To pull the ribs apart and expose the heart, retractors are placed on the divided breastbone and screwed apart. As they open the chest, the heart can be seen beating beneath the smooth sac which surrounds it. To confirm the diagnosis, the surgeon slits the pericardium and looks for the defects which X-rays and catheterization have told him will be there. In this case, he sees from the state of the heart that he has to deal with a hole between the main chambers.

Before the heart is touched the patient is given heparin through the needle in his arm vein. The blood-pressure recorder is placed in the right artery and the heart and brain tracing are checked.

One by one the plastic lines from the machine are prepared and fitted with the steel nozzles or cannulae. One of these cannulae is placed in the left artery ready to return blood from the machine back into the body.

The surgeon now turns to the heart. In the left upper chamber he inserts several stitches and draws them tight. Then he incises between the threads and pushes a cannula into the wall of the chamber, pulling the stitches round it to prevent blood leakage. One of the two pumps has now been tied into the circuit; it will take blood from the left chamber and pump it back into the leg artery.

The surgeon calls out, "Start left bypass," and an assistant switches on the pump which takes up slowly. Blood begins to drain into one of the plastic reservoirs, and as this fills the pump empties back into the leg artery.

"Begin cooling now," the surgeon announces.

The switch is moved to "Cold" and the unit outside the theatre begins to pump cold water through the tall cylinder, bringing its temperature down gradually from 98.4 degrees Fahrenheit. The surgeon gives a look at the control unit on the pump to see if the cooling has started and then begins to tie in the right pump of the machine to the right atrium and ventricle.

First he places stitches to hold the steel end of the tube and then nicks the right upper chamber of the heart, inserts the tube end and pulls the stitches tight. A stab incision is made in the right lower chamber and another cannula is placed in the entrance to the pulmonary artery.

Now the pressure in the arteries falls as cooling checks the flow of blood. The right-hand pump has begun to take over the circulation of blood through the lungs, and the body temperature is dropping rapidly.

With the temperature more than 15 degrees below normal the heart shows signs of fibrillation—the spasmodic twitching of its lower chambers which the hypothermia surgeon once dreaded. But with two pumps looking after the blood flow the surgeon does not worry, and the temperature still falls.

The temperature gauge reads 20 degrees Centigrade—68 degrees F.—and the pattern of waves on the machine recording the brain signals suddenly changes. Instead of the tall, ragged lines the signals have straightened out—and no electrical echoes at all come from the brain. The heart still beats, slowly but regularly, writing long drawn-out signals on the electrocardiograph.

But, as the temperature falls still further, the heart, too, changes its rhythm and its beat becomes tired and ponderous. Down and down goes the temperature gauge until it stands at 50 degrees F. The heart is making its last efforts to beat, but at that level of cooling it, too, gives up and falls flaccid into its hollow in the chest.

"Stop the pumps," demands the surgeon, and the machine suddenly comes to a halt. The pen recorders are switched off, the artificial respiration is suspended. And the surgeon notes the exact minute on the clock at which everything has been cooled into silence.

The boy on the table is dead—clinically a cadaver. His heart and blood have ceased to move; his lungs are lying still; his brain has gone out like a light in a dark cellar. He has been put into a sort of Rip van Winkle sleep to be roused with a new heart.

Forty-five minutes. That is the deadline which the surgeon has allowed himself to make good the heart's faults and end this period of suspended animation. Quickly he clamps off the main vessels threading in and out of the heart to prevent air lock; the tube nozzle is pulled out of the right heart chamber through which he will cut to get at the hole in the middle wall. But before this he drains the heart of its blood and it sags and collapses like a pricked balloon.

"Five minutes," says the voice of the man on the pump.

The heart lies dry and open. Through the long slit in the right chamber the hole can be seen in the wall. An easy one which can be closed with silk thread. He places the first sutures, drawing them together and tying each as he goes to add strength to the repair.

"Twenty minutes."

The surgeon ties all but the last stitch in the defect. An assistant loosens some of the clamps and the left pump is given a turn to drive blood through the left to the right heart. This displaces air through the small hole left in the defect.

"Thirty minutes."

The last stitch is tied. All that remains is the sewing of the long cut in the right heart chamber. Again this is done in stages so that air can be driven out of the right side.

At the pump, the operator prepares to start rewarming by throwing the heat-exchanger switch to "Hot". The cannulae

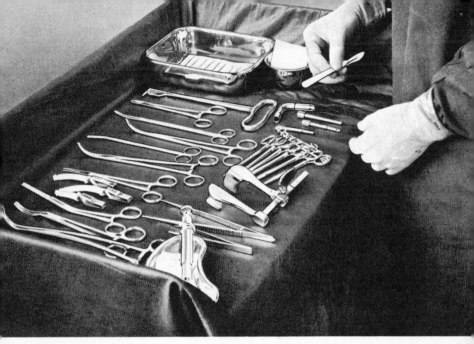

A heart surgeon holds a modern scalpel with detachable blade over a table which shows the array of forceps, rib retractors and other instruments used in heart operations

A British team at Brompton Hospital demonstrates to foreign surgeons a method of repairing a hole in the upper heart chambers by cooling the patient's blood until the heart stops. Blood is pumped from the great veins through a cooling coil immersed in an icebath and then returned to the body

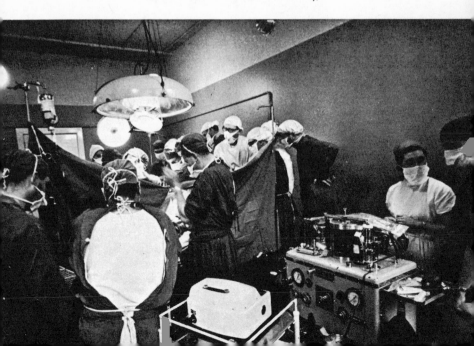

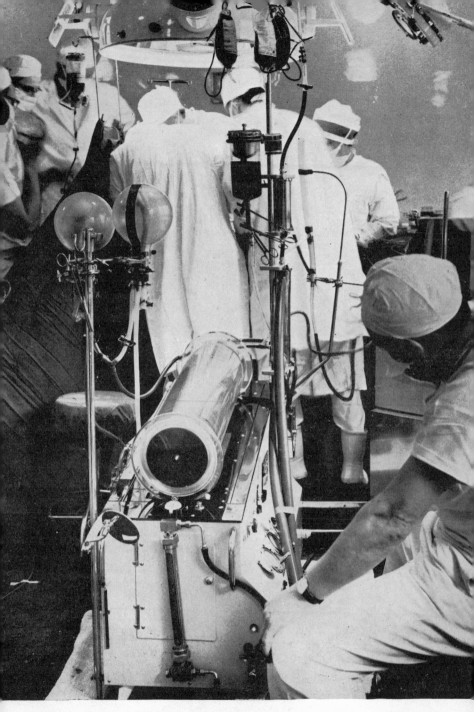

The Melrose–NEP machine is seen in the foreground, with its plastic cylinder spinning to keep the patient's blood saturated with oxygen while surgeons operate on the heart. The plastic tubes bring spent blood from the heart, push it through the revolving cylinder and then pump it back into an artery are replaced, and the surgeon gives the order: "Start the pumps."

For a few minutes the pumps run without heating the blood, and then the warming process is started.

Quickly the temperature begins to rise, and the voice of an assistant calls out: 13.5 . . . 16.1 . . . 18.5 . . . At 20 degrees C.— 65 F.—the brain trace begins to scribble the familiar waves, and the electrocardiograph picks up the currents from the heart.

As the temperature climbs the heart trace breaks from the slow, measured pace into a frantic scrawl which tells the theatre staff that it is fibrillating. They wait for a few minutes—the pumps are still in charge—to see if it reverts spontaneously to normal rhythm. If not, they may have to shock it back into its stride. But this time, as is usual with children, the heart finds its own beat and the staff relax.

The operation is all but over. When the temperature has reached into the nineties the pumps are stopped, the right first and then the left; the tubes are withdrawn from the heart and the leg artery. All the vessels are delicately repaired and the chest is closed.

The boy is wheeled out of the theatre. The surgeon and his staff take off the masks and smocks which they have worn for five hours. The day after tomorrow they have the same ritual to go through . . . and a queue of a few hundred patients who are waiting their turn to be placed in this nether world of hypothermia while their hearts are patched.

The drug company, Allen and Hanbury Ltd. made a film of the Drew technique. The Peripatetic Correspondent of the *Lancet* was invited to watch the filmed operation on a seven-year-old boy at a London hospital. It lasted eight hours, and he described the imposing variety of operating procedures which the surgeon and his staff carried out on the patient, a young boy.

Two days later he went to see the boy in his ward.

"Hullo, old chap!" he said. "I wanted to see how you are getting on; I was at your operation."

"You were?" said the boy. "That operation," he went on, "they pricked my finger; it still hurts."

Although hypothermia gained its impetus from men who wanted to tackle the long queues of heart cripples, surgeons in other fields adopted cold-sleep when they met emergencies. Since it slowed the heart and blood pressure it could save life dramatically by arresting massive haemorrhages.

Neither Mrs. Ellen Moore nor her child would be alive today were it not for hypothermia. This pretty, golden-haired woman of 22 was escorting her mother to a bus stop in a New-castle street at 2.45 on the afternoon of the 4th of May, 1956. She pushed a pram with her 18-month-old child in it and the two women had been discussing the child which earlier that day doctors had told Mrs. Moore she was expecting. The young mother did not see the 30-foot tree trunk which rolled off the lorry and sent her spinning against a wall. A passer-by dialled 999 for an ambulance, but the crowd which collected believed the woman to be dead.

Two ambulance men arrived in a few minutes, and within half an hour Mrs. Moore lay in the neuro-surgical unit of the Newcastle General Hospital. There, the surgeon-in-charge, Mr. George Rowbotham, saw she had severe injuries on the left side of the head. She showed all the signs of a brain haemorr-hage. The surgeon noted the deep coma, the large pupils which did not react to bright light and the lack of reflexes.

Should they operate to attempt to remove the blood clot which they suspected? Before the surgeon had time to decide; before he could perform the spinal puncture which would tell him there was a brain haemorrhage, Mrs. Moore's tempera-ture began to rise perilously. Though they kept the ward cool the thermometer climbed steadily from 2 a.m. until it stood eight hours later at 105.5 F.

The staff had seen cases like this before. Invariably they spelled death in three days. Hypothermia seemed to offer the only hope of saving the mother. They knew about the unborn child, eight weeks old, and the fact that cooling had never been used before on a pregnant woman. They resolved to take a chance.

To prevent shivering and help pull down the temperature, they opened a vein and gave Mrs. Moore chlorpromazine and promethazine, two of the drugs which Laborit had used in his Lytic Cocktail, and pethidine as an analgesic. They then sponged her with iced water and placed ice packs round her body while cold air was blown over her bed. By 6 p.m. seven hours after the hypothermia treatment started, the temperature had dropped to 86 F., though the level of consciousness remained the same.

The case of what the Press called the Sleeping Beauty roused wide interest. The hospital issued a bulletin which said: "She reacted to no known kind of stimuli. In an attempt to save her life all the newer methods of medical science were invoked, and by means of cooling anaesthesia she was put into a virtual state of hibernation.

"She was left in hibernation for seven days, during which her temperature was down to 86 F. This method tided her over the most dangerous phase of her illness and probably saved her life, because her temperature at the time was rising to a dangerous level."

Much was made at the time of the doctors' dilemma; they had to save the child, it was said. The surgeons really fought to save both mother and child. When they believed that the cerebral bleeding had ceased, they brought her temperature slowly back to normal. Even this did not pull her out of the deep coma in which she had lain since arriving at the hospital, and another four long weeks of nursing and feeding her with liquid food and vitamins went by before she opened her eyes in Ward 27. Then Mrs. Moore, in the words of the surgeon and his three staff, "became one of the most difficult problems that the medical service ever had to deal with." She found it impossible to lie still and ruined dozens of bed sheets by pulling and biting them. Nor would she allow any of the doctors or nurses to come near or examine her.

Mr. Linton Snaith, Senior Obstetrician and Gynaecologist, had assumed that Mrs. Moore was pregnant from the clinic report, though not until the 10th of August could he confirm the report and say that the child still lived. Neither Snaith nor the hospital staff could approach Mrs. Moore to examine her in the early stages of her treatment. "She showed extreme cerebral irritability, and was uncontrollable if any attempt at physical examination was made," Mr. Snaith wrote of the case.

The pregnancy seemed to be proceeding normally, though the doctors were worried about the effect of hypothermia on the child. For seven days, in the ninth week of pregnancy, the mother had been cooled. But medical evidence suggested that the child would withstand the low temperatures, and the doctors therefore expected a normal birth. On the 18th of November, six-and-a-half months after entering the hospital, Mrs. Moore's baby was born and the delivery gave little trouble. It was a boy, 7 lb. 12 oz. in weight and perfectly normal. Stephen Moore became the first baby to be born by virtue of hypothermia, and today is none the worse for the experience. Mrs. Moore's condition improved greatly within a few weeks of the operation.

Brain surgeons have adopted hypothermia in routine work and for the type of emergency which faced the doctors at Newcastle. Cooling reduces the blood flow and the pressure on the brain and this helps the surgeon in dealing with damaged arteries, brain clots and bleeding.

15

Back from the Dead

EVEN the doctors at the Harvard Medical School found it difficult to believe. Here they had an old man who should have died more than two days ago, but who looked like recovering. For fifty-two hours, and they had timed it to the minute, his heart had not helped itself in any way, yet it still beat strongly and etched a regular pattern on the electro-cardiogram trace.

On the 28th of September, 1952, the 65-year-old man had come into the medical school, a hopeless invalid with a wobbling heart which had been crippled with coronary disease eight years before. His medical card read: Congestive heart failure and heart block.

Heart block was the condition which interested one of the surgeons at the Boston medical school. Dr. Paul Zoll, like many other cardiac experts, thought that when the heart's clockwork began to run down he might succeed in devising a method of rewinding it.

The heart has its own metronome which regulates its explosive muscular action. Not so long ago, cardiologists believed this beat was regulated by nerve cells. But nowadays, with better instruments, doctors know that the pacemaking impulses rise in special bundles of muscle on the heart itself. High up, on the right receiving chamber, lies a knot of this muscle which triggers off the electrical impulse which sweeps through the two atria like a spark along a powder train, causing them to squeeze blood into the ventricles. With perfect timing, the spark initiated in the atria ripples down through a coil of muscles to another knot of pacemaking tissue in the ventricles. This impulse makes the two main pumping chambers clench like a powerful fist and drive blood out to the arteries and the lungs. First, the atria; then, eight-hundredths of a second later, the ventricles. And the pacemaker will keep them firing 2,500 million times in the average life. Until it breaks down.

The pacemaker can run amok for two reasons. The muscle of the heart may degenerate when a coronary artery blocks and stops feeding them. The trelliswork of muscle ceases to conduct the impulses which trigger the lower chambers. With so much heart surgery today, these conducting muscles are often cut and while they heal the surgical scar leaves a gap which the heart current cannot leap. The heart has, so to speak, blown a fuse; the ventricles are isolated and left to work on their own.

Fortunately, the ventricles will keep going independently of the atria—but much slower. While the upper chambers beat at 70 to the minute, the lower ones can manage about 40. With its main pumps out of phase and partially crippled, the heart ceases to do its full job of driving blood through the body. And the patient with heart block soon feels this blood starvation in terms of breathlessness, dizziness and chest trouble. Sometimes the heart will fail completely for a minute or two; the bloodline to the brain is cut; and the patient blacks out, to recover only when the ventricles take up their irregular beat again.

No one had devised a method of coping with heart block. Bigelow, to whom we owe so many ideas in cardiac work, suggested using electric shocks to keep the heart beats in phase, but had not tried himself with patients.

At Harvard, Zoll and a group of young doctors had taken the matter further. With animals they discovered that electric shocks passed to terminals placed in the food tract and stuck to the chest did keep failing hearts beating rhythmically. But they had yet to prove the method on patients with heart block.

They had tried in only one case—a 75-year-old-man who had suffered from heart block for two years. But it seemed that repeated injections of heart stimulants had caused the organ to fail before they tested their apparatus.

Now they had the chance to use their pacemaker on a man who was in the last stages of heart failure. For six days they had kept him alive with repeated injections of drugs. But their recordings revealed that the two main chambers were beating at half the normal pace; and often, in fact, the heart stood still for anything up to a minute.

The doctors attached the pacemaker which Zoll had devised. One needle was thrust under the skin at the apex of the heart; another on the skin surface at the fourth rib space. These were connected to an electricity supply which could deliver shocks lasting two-thousandths of a second, 50 to 100 times a minute. On the electrocardiogram these shocks came up plainly, proving that the machine was maintaining heart rhythm.

For the next three days they watched the heart, switching on the pacemaker only when the ventricles came to a halt.

At 12.30 p.m. on the 7th of October, the heart failed and the doctors switched over to the pacemaker. At ninety shocks to the minute the heart began to beat steadily and showed no signs of stopping so long as impulses were fed to it by the machine. For fifty-two hours the artificial timekeeping device fired current into the lower chambers of the heart to keep them contracting—without once receiving help from the heart itself! Several times they switched off the current; on each occasion the heart died. From studying heart traces, Zoll and his colleagues could state that only the outside stimulation was driving the ventricles.

In the afternoon of the 9th of October, the ventricles took up a spontaneous beat of 44 a minute and the pace-maker was shut off; the electrodes were removed two days later;

and the patient began to sit up, to be told that he had been living on electric shocks for five days. He seemed none the worse for the experience and left the hospital not long afterwards, his heart still beating regularly.

Zoll's method had several drawbacks. To apply shocks to the heart through thick layers of flesh, the ribs and the heart sac, he had to work with high voltages which sent the chest muscles into spasm and often caused burns. There had to be a better way—and two colleagues of Zoll found it at Harvard. They took the problem to Dr. Frederick Vanderschmidt, of the Massachusetts Institute of Technology, and he designed a small transistor battery which would feed shocks of half a volt directly into the heart. The two surgeons opened the chests of animals and stitched the positive and negative leads of the generator into the upper chambers of the heart. By placing them on the spot where the heart initiated its own beat, the generator picked up these tiny natural shocks, amplified them and passed them on to the ventricles. The Harvard pair proved that this type of pacemaker would steady an unruly heart for days at a time. This method had the advantage of keeping the upper and lower chambers in phase. But again Lillehei came up with the suggestion which did much to solve the problem. His hundreds of operations had taught him that heart block followed in a big proportion of hole-in-the-heart patients, however carefully the surgeon might avoid cutting the conducting muscle bundle. Surely, said the Minneapolis surgeon, we can stitch electrodes directly on to the heart, lead them out through the chest and run a pulsed current through them.

He and two colleagues, William L. Weirich and Vincent L. Gott, first proved the principle in animals. Then, with patients whose hearts went into block during or after operations, they saved many lives by tying pacemakers into the muscle of the ventricles. For the negative lead, they took a length of silver-plated and braided copper wire no thicker than their suturing silk. This, they implanted in the wall of the right ventricle and ran out through the chest as they closed it. The other lead they sewed under the skin opposite the apex of the heart. Then they pushed just under two and a half volts through the leads on to the heart. Their first patient, a child whose heart went into block during an operation, was successfully treated by the new method on the 30th of January, 1957. In the months which followed this case, Lillehei and his group saved eighteen patients with heart block. Only one of these died—and that happened when the chest lead was accidentally removed.

In Britain, too, doctors had developed pacemaking equipment which kept the heart alive by shocks applied directly to its muscle. Three doctors at St. George's Hospital, London, built a pacemaker for a few pounds and used it to save a 68-year-old woman with heart block.

In a few years the pacemaker became standard, sitting beside the other instruments near the operating table. Not only do surgeons use it for patients who develop heart block; it will tide the heart over other types of failure. Most of the present-day pacemakers are implanted under the skin and fed by batteries which can be carried around with the patient. Some of them need to be charged every so often in the way that radio or car batteries have to be boosted.

Harold Maskell was typical of those people who owed their lives to an artificial timekeeper which sustained the beat of their hearts. I met him, in July, 1960, when he came into St. George's Hospital to have his heart battery charged for another seven days. The ruddy-cheeked, grey-haired pensioner sat up in bed and told me how fit he had felt since surgeons, eleven weeks before, had planted an electric pacemaker just below his heart. The dizzy spells and blackouts which had plagued him for years had gone and he could now walk around without fear that he would pass out and not recover.

Harold's story was like hundreds of others: heart block had

forced him to lead a life free of exertion or excitement which, doctors told him, might have induced heart failure. But at 65 his heart seemed good for several more years, if it could be kept beating rhythmically. At the London teaching hospital the surgeons were trying out a new pacemaker designed by Swedish doctor Rune Elmquist and Mr. Maskell agreed to an operation to embed the pacemaker in his chest and link it with his heart.

The Swedish designer had worked on the principle that an electric stimulator ought to be buried in the body; those attached to the outside of the chest might be pulled off, with death as the sequel; they also handicapped the patient in his movements. His answer looked like a pocket watch made of plastic, which Elmquist chose because it produced no reaction in the body. Into the plastic case he fitted a voltage generator with two small insulated wires which could be stuck and stitched into the ventricles. Also in the plastic pacemaker was a tiny battery to feed the voltage pulses into the wires. Since the pacemaker could not be removed every time the battery ran down, it was designed to be recharged by induction from a power source outside the body.

So Harold had an operation in which the lower part of his chest was opened and two leads were sewn into the wall of the heart; the pacemaker, just under four inches in diameter, was placed under a thick fold of skin below the heart. Switched on, the pacemaker kept the ventricles pumping at seventy beats a minute, and Harold had no further trouble with his heart. Every week though, he made a ten-mile journey from his home in Enfield to the hospital to have another seven-day charge of electricity to keep his battery and his heart going. Now, Elmquist has designed a pacemaker with a mercury battery which will last three years.

In another British hospital, the Queen Elizabeth, Birmingham, two medical men and a technician took the pacemaking technique a step further by inventing a machine which lay under the skin but could be charged from a battery carried round by the patient. Their apparatus worked on the principle of the car coil where a primary circuit induces pulses into a secondary winding. The secondary coil, the size of a wrist watch and embedded in nylon, could be placed in the chest muscle opposite the heart with its two terminals running directly to the heart chambers. This secondary coil received its current from a pulse generator placed on the chest at the level of the inner coil. The master generator was made to deliver up to nine volts and pulses between 30 and 100 a minute, so that the patient could regulate his own heart beat and the surgeon could bring the ventricle rhythm into line with the pace of the upper chambers.

One of the emergencies which faces every surgeon at some moment in his career is heart arrest. The anaesthetist suddenly notices that the blood pressure is falling, the pulse has faded and the patient's colour has assumed a blue tint. The main cause of operating theatre deaths, cardiac arrest, seems para-doxically enough to be increasing as the apparel of modern surgery becomes more refined.

The indictments have touched anaesthesia. One eminent British pharmacologist pointed out just before the war that progress in anaesthesia appeared to have increased the risk of death on the table from heart failure. "The fact," said Professor A. J. Clark, "that deaths under anaesthesia are increasing rather than decreasing indicates that we are far from having attained perfection." But other factors undoubtedly contribute: a damaged heart, or even nervous apprehension are among them.

At one time when the heart stopped few surgeons would have attempted to revive it. Today, the surgeon who fails to attempt to bring a dead heart to life is guilty of negligence.

Some surgeons have worked on hearts for as long as twenty-four hours before they started to beat . . . and kept on beating.

The modern operator is equipped to cope with the stopped heart, and expects to save one in every two cases who "die" during operations. As long ago as 1899, the German surgeon, Johann Prus, showed that the heart could be massaged back into activity. He, himself, had practised the technique on animals by exposing the heart and kneading the ventricles in his hands. But only in recent years has the importance of speed been brought home to the surgeon. When the heart stops and blood-flow to the brain comes to a standstill, the higher cells quickly begin to perish, and the surgeon has no more than three minutes to restore the blood supply by massaging the heart.

The heart surgeon only worries about cardiac arrest if he is operating without a machine. And since he is working on the heart the massage which keeps it going is simple. The surgeon who is involved elsewhere in the body has a more difficult task. He must open the heart, normally through the fourth rib space, and then begin to resuscitate it.

The first thing he does is squeeze the heart by taking it between the heel of the hand and his closed fingers and compressing it firmly but gently about sixty times a minute. Two hands are better than one and many surgeons use the flat of both hands because this does less damage and is less tiring. If the heart then refuses to take up its own beat he might try stimulating it either by injecting drugs or by electric shock. In the thirties, the principle of shocking the heart back into life was tried experimentally by Dr. D. S. Hooker and Dr. Carl Wiggers in America, and found successful.

It fell to one of the great modern pioneers of heart surgery to demonstrate for the first time that the dead could be brought back to life by heart masssage coupled with electric-shock treatment. Professor Claude S. Beck, head of the department of Cardiovascular Surgery of the Western Reserve University, Cleveland, has a reputation as a man who does not yield easily to death. To him the extinction of life becomes a fact only when the surgeon and his staff have exhausted themselves and their armoury of instruments in trying to beat death.

Beck, who initiated many new concepts in heart surgery, appreciated before the majority of his colleagues that the factors which led to instability and death in the heart were reversible; that they had their origin in the electrical impulses which keep the heart beating regularly and therefore in the supply of oxygen to the organ. If shocks arising in the heart mechanism itself could electrocute the heart could not the same mechanism be used to restart it? Hooker, Wiggers and Beck himself had done it experimentally. Beck determined that he would give patients who "died" on the table a second chance by moving the electric shock equipment into the operating theatre.

Five times he tried to resuscitate hearts which had failed before he could report his first successful case. In the winter of 1947 a boy had come into Beck's hospital in Cleveland for a chest operation. Fourteen years of age, he had a "funnel chest"; his heart was displaced and he complained of breathlessness when he took exercise.

Beck did the chest operation, during which the heart raced for forty-five minutes at more than twice its normal rhythm. When he came to close the wound, the trouble began . . . the heart which had steadied during surgery suddenly stopped, the blood pressure sagged, the pulse and breathing came to a standstill.

Immediately, the surgeon re-opened the chest and began to massage the heart, his assistants pumping stimulant drugs into a vein and giving the boy oxygen through an anaesthetic tube. For thirty-five minutes Beck continued to squeeze the heart, until it began to flutter weakly and uselessly. When Beck had massaged the heart for another ten minutes and felt that a shock might restart it, he placed the two terminals of his electrical equipment over the ventricles and applied a shock to the heart. Still it did not respond.

Into the right auricle the surgeon pushed a hypodermic needle and injected a stimulant. For some time he kept massaging the heart and then decided to try another series of shocks. This time, the surgeon noted that the heart had begun to beat, feebly and rapidly—but regularly. As he continued the massage for five minutes it became obvious that beneath his hands, the heart was beating of its own accord. From its swift pace—175 beats a minute—it gradually steadied and grew stronger, until there was no more need to watch it. The boy recovered with no damage to his brain or any other organ.

Beck had established the technique; had shown that a heart could be kept alive, and the circulation, too, while surgeons did their best to salvage patients with electric shock treatment.

Beck did more than practise resuscitation in his own hospitals; he preached it wherever he went . . . at medical meetings, to surgeons, physicians, students and even to first-aid men. The suggestion that every operating theatre should have its revival kit came from him. In the year that he carried out his famous case he attended the Detroit Symposium on Cardiovascular Surgery and, in forthright terms, told fellow-surgeons that they ought to train their teams in reviving dead hearts.

"I would like to say," he told them, "that any normal heart can be made to beat again if properly handled. I think it is up to us surgeons to see to it that we do know how to do it properly.

"I want to mention the responsibility that we surgeons have to society for resuscitation. This knowledge of resuscitation has been in existence for a good many years, and, if I may say so, I think we have been a bit derelict in picking it up. Just within our family, I would like to say that we really should not operate on a patient unless we know how to resuscitate his heart if it should stop.

"I don't think we are doing the right thing for our patient unless we have knowledge of the resuscitation procedures. I think it is a crime for a surgeon to walk away from the operating table, the patient dying, without doing anything. If I were on a jury in a court and had to make a decision about the responsibility for the death of a patient with a previously normal heart who died on the operating table, I would have to vote against the surgeon.

"There is no excuse, it seems to me, for a surgeon not knowing how to resuscitate a heart. Courses have been established in various parts of the country to teach surgeons and anaesthetists how to do it. It is exceedingly simple. We ought to avail ourselves of those courses."

Today, most operating theatres have a machine standing by which will generate a current of 220 volts at sixty cycles a second. When the heart muscle begins to recover its tone the surgeon can then pass a shock through it for about a quarter of a second. If one jolt of current does not trigger off heart action, he can then try a series of six or eight quick shocks at lower voltages.

Even among the highly-disciplined staff of an operating theatre heart arrest causes consternation, and one prominent surgeon estimates that it takes half a minute to start the resuscitation drill. Even so, some strange cases are recorded of people dropping dead outside the operating theatres and being revived without signs of brain damage.

It was just on lunch time eight days before the Christmas of 1954. Three men were working together in the darkroom of the Lutheran Deaconess Hospital in Chicago, developing X-ray films, when in the blacked-out room two of them heard a thud, heavy and so unexpected that it took several seconds to grope for the lights and switch them on.

The young X-ray technician lay on the floor where he had fallen and his colleagues could see that he was not breathing or moving. One of them ran for the radiologist, Dr. Frank Hussey, who hurried in, felt the man's pulse and ordered adrenaline to inject into the heart to try to stimulate it into action. While they waited for the drug, another doctor, Joel Knudson, was summoned and began to give artificial respiration.

The 24-year-old technician was laid on his back, his shoulders propped up while Dr. Knudson took his arms and alternately stretched them above his head and flexed them across his chest to keep air filling his lungs. Passing the X-ray room at the time was Dr. C. David Brown of the surgical department. Quickly he filled a syringe with adrenaline and emptied it into the heart. But the doctors felt that the short needle had not gone beyond the pericardium—and the heart showed no signs of life.

There was no pulse; the stethoscope picked up no heart sounds; no breathing. And yet the technician had come through two stiff medical tests in June and October, the first as a naval officer and the second for an insurance company. These had thrown no doubts on his health and fitness.

The two doctors consulted each other quickly. Clinically, the man was dead. They had nothing to lose if they opened his chest and massaged his heart.

Speed was essential. Since he had fallen minutes had ticked away; and both doctor and surgeon realized they had between three and four minutes to start his heart before death began to take over the brain cells. They did not consider moving him to an operating theatre.

Brown had a stub-bladed knife in his pocket. With frantic discipline they bared the young technician's chest and the

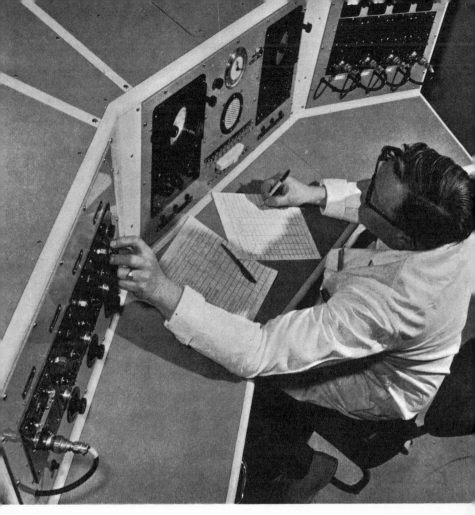

A doctor monitors the condition of a patient undergoing heart surgery with an "electronic brain" placed outside the operating theatre. The dials indicate the patient's blood pressure, temperature, brain activity and biochemical alterations of the blood

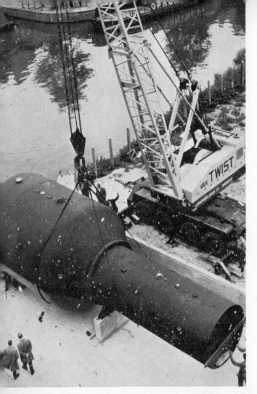

The bottom photograph shows a Dutch team of surgeons operating inside a pressure chamber equipped as a surgical theatre. By pumping up the chamber to three times the normal atmospheric pressure the surgeons can saturate the patient with oxygen and give the body an oxygen "bank" while they stop the heart. This hyperpression method of heart surgery was devised by Professor Ite Boerema, of Amsterdam University. The original hyperpression experiments were conducted in a regulation naval decompression chamber, which the Royal Dutch Navy lent the professor and which can be seen at left

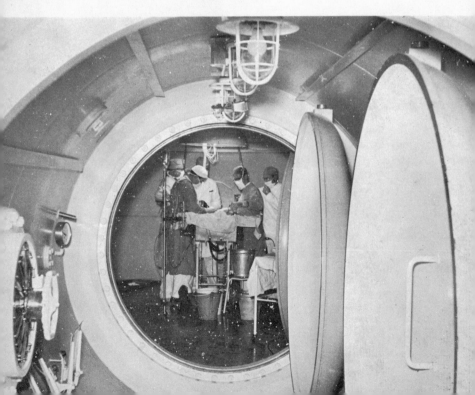

surgeon drew the knife deeply between the fourth and fifth ribs, cutting through into the chest cavity. They prised a rib apart—and there lay the heart, still and small, stopped in the moment of contraction. The circulation had halted, for no blood seeped from the wound they had made. There was a danger of sepsis, but in such a life-and-death case the doctors had to take the risk.

A third man had looked in by chance and joined the team. Dr. George F. Schroeder assembled the oxygen apparatus, put a mask over the man's face while Brown started to massage the heart. Sixty seconds of rhythmic squeezing and the organ quivered into life. But not the normal, steady beat. The heart was squirming and writhing hopelessly.

For a few moments they stopped massaging . . . just long enough to get the technician round the dark-room maze and on to a surgical trolley. Even on the way to the operating theatre the doctors still carried on with massage and oxygen treatment. Four minutes had gone by before they had opened the chest; another minute had elapsed while they massaged and brought a little life back into the heart. Was there still a chance?

They laid the man on an operating table, slipped an anaesthetic tube down his throat and began to pump oxygen into his lungs to keep them inflated and recharge the blood.

Another three minutes.

Now, six surgical staff had gathered round the figure on the table, taking it in turns to massage the heart. It seemed futile.

They decided to try shocking the heart back into normal rhythm. The hospital had no shock equipment but another hospital sent theirs over by ambulance. A groan went up when the machine short-circuited. They called the University of Illinois hospital. It was not feasible, said the chief anaesthetist, to bring the electric-shock machine over. Time was too short.

The anaesthetist suggested stopping the heart with a chemical injection and restarting it with a neutralizing substance.

They stopped the heart—but could not jolt it into action. More massage only brought back the fibrillation. Again they tried; again they got the same result. The third time they resolved to let the heart stand still for half a minute. They stopped it . . . counted out the thirty seconds . . . and then began pumping the heart with their hands.

Miraculously, the four chambers began to beat, slowly at first and then with the solid rhythm which told them that they need no longer worry.

They looked at the clock in the operating theatre. Just after 3.15 p.m. The heart had been out of action for a hundred and thirty-five minutes . . . and had come back to life again.

They placed the technician in an oxygen tent. The heart was bounding at almost double the normal rate; his breathing was fast and thin. But twenty-four hours later he sat up and talked to his parents when they came to visit him. He still remained hazy about what had happened at the developing table in the dark-room, but three days later his mind had cleared. The doctors, who might have expected some memory disorder, found the man completely recovered mentally.

In a fortnight, the young technician was out of bed and walking about the ward. Twenty-two days after he had "died" he went home by car. Periodic checks revealed his heart to be normal; he skated, played baseball and did his job for two years after the incident without losing a day on account of illness.

But he is only one of the strange cases of people who have been snatched from death by resourceful surgeons. Claude Beck, one of the first men to tackle coronary artery disease by surgery, believes that the heart fails in many instances through some small instability; that death should not win without a tussle. This case, which he described, is typical of the way in which death may be reversed.

The doctor had come to University Hospitals in Cleveland for a check-up. He was 65, still practising as a family doctor in the city, but for some months had suffered from chronic indigestion. On the 21st of June, 1955, he felt violent pains over his heart which the usual treatment with stomach powder did nothing to relieve. He diagnosed an attack of angina pectoris and made a date at the hospital for the next morning. There, at 11.30 a.m. they ran off an electrocardiogram and did a few other routine tests. The doctor dressed and prepared to leave the hospital.

At 12.55 p.m., as he walked through the entrance, he collapsed and lay for about a minute before the hospital staff carried him to the emergency operating theatre near where he had fallen.

By the theatre clock it was 12.57. The physician had no pulse; he did not breathe; his face and hands were blue; the surgeons could hear no heart sounds.

Beck and two colleagues, Elden C. Weckesser and Frank M. Barry, first gave him artificial respiration and oxygen through a face mask. The heart did not respond when they punctured it with a needle. "The man was dead," said the doctors in their report, published by the *Journal of the American Medical Association.*

Four minutes after he collapsed they slit the chest open between the fourth and fifth ribs, which they drew back to expose the heart. One of the surgeons placed a hand beneath the heart, and without giving himself time to open the pericardium began to massage the heart against the breastbone. Even through the sac surrounding the heart they could observe that the heart had begun to twist and writhe in fibrillation.

Eight minutes after the man "died" they slipped a breathing tube into his throat and gave him oxygen through this. The colour started to flow back into his cheeks and skin, and the staff noticed that, every now and again, he tried to breathe. For two more minutes one of the surgeons emptied the heart by squeezing it slowly and rhythmically with his hand. Beck then tried to shock the heart into its normal beat by placing two spade electrodes on the lower chambers and passing a high voltage through them for two seconds. But still the heart fluttered, and they had to keep the massage going.

For another fifteen minutes they pumped the heart. Three more shocks still failed to jerk it into action on its own. Then the surgeons realized what had gone wrong. The gauze covering on the electrodes was dry; no current had passed through the heart. Quickly they steeped the electrodes in salt water and applied them to the heart. For two seconds they held them there; the fluttering pulse stopped; and the heart picked up its beat.

When they had put the physician to bed under an oxygen tent they looked at the electrocardiogram which had been taken that morning. Clearly it proved the physician to have had a coronary thrombosis a short time before.

The morning after he "died" the doctor responded to questions and by midday was speaking a few words. But it took two days of careful nursing before he spoke and moved properly. When he left hospital after eleven days he was quite normal—except for a memory lapse covering thirty-six hours before the incident. After convalescence he was well enough to go back to work.

In their report Beck and his colleagues compared heart failure to a car with its ignition turned off, or a stopped clock. "The heart wants to beat and often it needs only a second chance," they said. The vast majority of deaths from heart failure occurred through electrical instability; probably one in ten were caused by muscle damage.

Beck's report contained one main argument: Not only doctors and surgeons should be trained in reviving hearts which had stopped; the public, too, might save those people who dropped dead in the street or on the golf course. Medical authorities might provide life-saving kits in certain areas so that prompt action could be taken. The Beck report ended with these words: "The veil of mystery is being lifted from heart conditions, and the dead are being brought back to life."

Two British physicians repeated Beck's feat of saving a man who had suffered a coronary. A 39-year-old Pole owes his life to the speed with which the two doctors acted when they picked him up unconscious in the casualty department of King's College Hospital, London. The Pole, a cleaner, came in for treatment on the night of the 6th of February, 1960, and joined a queue in the waiting-room. Quarter of an hour later he had collapsed.

The casualty officer, Dr. Paul Brass, and the house physician, Dr. Robert Kendell, had him carried to the nearest examination cubicle where they tried to revive him with an intravenous injection. But a few minutes later his heart stopped; the doctors made a quick diagnosis of heart failure due to coronary thrombosis. It was then 8.42 p.m.

Quickly they cut away his clothes and opened the chest along the fifth rib space, at the same time slipping an anaesthetic tube into his windpipe. No bleeding came from the wound they had made, and both noticed why; the heart stood still. Without troubling to open the pericardium they began massage to keep the brain alive; they also gave oxygen to keep the lungs inflated.

Slowly the Pole's colour returned, and five minutes after they had begun massage they injected a stimulant directly into the left heart chamber. Within a minute the man started breathing and his heart moved weakly. But the heart did not resume its normal beat; instead it began to twitch spasmodically and the doctors went on with massage.

For nearly half an hour they kept pumping the heart—until

an anaesthetist arrived with electrical apparatus to shock the heart. Dipped in salt solution, the cloth-bound electrodes were placed across the lower chambers and four shocks were tried. Still the heart would not come to life.

Forty minutes after the heart had failed, a double shock of 200 volts jolted it into life again, and this time it maintained its rhythm.

The doctors found later that the man had suffered from a coronary attack the previous year, and had spent six weeks in their own hospital. It was one of the rare cases of heart revival following a coronary. On the 5th of April the man left hospital to convalesce—with only a memory lapse covering the four days from February 6th to 10th as a result of his experience.

Surgeons were still not satisfied with the massage techniques which involved exposing the heart. They were time-consuming, and might leave the patient not only with permanent muscle damage but with infection from an unsterile operation.

Dr. William B. Kouwenhoven and three colleagues at the Johns Hopkins Medical School had already invented equipment to apply a shock to the heart through the chest wall. But they soon realized that this instrument must be used within minutes of heart standstill, so Kouwenhoven looked round for methods of keeping the heart alive to give the apparatus the best chance of restarting the organ.

Several surgeons and physicians had tried before him to revive patients without resorting to surgery. Two British doctors had found in the thirties that rocking patients from head to toe kept up their blood pressure; another pair of British anaesthetists, Dr. Ernest Rainer and Dr. John Bullough, revived children who had "died" on the operating table by placing an arm beneath their knees and pumping their legs and buttocks against their chests.

Kouwenhoven practised several techniques on animals and

concluded that closed-chest massage coupled with his electric-shock treatment produced results as good as the surgical method. More interesting, when they came to try the Baltimore Method on patients whose hearts had given out on the operating table they discovered that they did not need their electrical equipment.

To carry out resuscitation, the Johns Hopkins group used only their hands and mouth-to-nose breathing. They laid the patient flat on his back on a firm surface. The heel of the right hand was placed on the breastbone with the left hand pressing on it. The heart could thus be compressed between the breastbone and the spine; the pericardium restricted movement of the heart to either side. In unconscious patients the rib cage had enough "give" to allow the surgeon to empty the heart and keep the lungs working. And where two people were performing resuscitation, one of them could breathe through the nose of the patient to fill the lungs with air.

Their first case, in July, 1959, was a woman, aged 35, who came into the Baltimore hospital with gall stones. Her heart stopped while she was going under the anaesthetic. One of the surgeons placed the heel of his hand over the woman's breastbone and pressed firmly and rhythmically on the chest at about sixty times a minute. Within two minutes the heart started beating again, and the operation was finished without further hitch.

At the beginning of 1960 the Baltimore doctors had another case where they coupled closed-chest massage with electric shock treatment. The man, 45 years of age, came into the casualty room with agonizing chest and arm pains. While they removed his clothes to examine him he fell dead on the floor. A quick check showed he had no pulse and was not breathing so the house physician immediately began vigorous massage while another doctor fixed electrocardiograph leads to his chest. The tracing showed the heart to be fibrillating wildly. Massage went on for twenty minutes while waiting for the shock equipment.

They passed two shocks through the chest—one to arrest the spasmodic heart action, and a second which triggered off normal heart beats. Heart tracings taken two hours later proved that the man had suffered a coronary attack. After treatment for the heart condition the man was discharged from hospital. But for the prompt action of the hospital staff he would have died: he was left with two hours missing from his memory, beginning from the moment that he collapsed.

The Baltimore Method has saved hundreds of lives in hospitals and outside. Now it has become part of first-aid training and with it the dead are being brought back to life.

16

The Surgeon Tackles Heart Artery Disease

ONE HEART disease has defied the surgeon just as it has baffled the physician since it made its first appearance on a death certificate. Now it ranks as the biggest single killer in the civilized world, carrying off literally millions of people every year. Coronary artery disease has attracted more medical attention than almost all the other diseases put together—and yet we seem no closer to a medical or surgical solution to its problems.

First described in 1912, coronary disease took some time to make its impact on the medical profession. All too often doctors labelled it as indigestion, rheumatism, influenza, pleurisy or fibrositis before they began to recognize it for what it really was. When they did, the disease quickly climbed the mortality tables, seeking its victims particularly among middle-aged and elderly men. Today, when fewer people are dying early from infectious illnesses, the medical statistician is confronted with the disquieting fact that coronary disease appears to be attacking young and active people in their forties—when the community needs them most. Recent statistics published by the World Health Organization prove that heart disease is the biggest threat to health in the well-fed Western countries.

The United States suffers most from heart disease, more than 700,000 people dying every year. To give some idea of the epidemic proportions of the disease, two out of every five male deaths in America are due to coronary and degenerative heart artery disease. In contrast, one in five women die from the condition. The W.H.O. survey, carried out in twenty-four countries, listed the countries with the highest incidence of coronary trouble. Just behind America comes Canada, with much the same death rate, White South Africans are next, then Australia, Finland and New Zealand. In Britain, just over a quarter of the men and one in seven of the women who die every year are victims of coronary disease. At the other end of the scale come France and Japan with an incidence six times less than the U.S.A. Unfortunately, the figures for the disease are still moving upwards. Much of the huge increase in the last fifteen years may be due to the improvements in diagnosis. In countries like the United States and Britain, where medical examination is more rigorous than in more backward countries, the experts expect to find a higher percentage of heart disease. As health services progress in other countries the incidence of coronary illness will probably rise dramatically, revealed by better detection methods. But much less obvious than the diagnosis of coronary disease are the reasons behind this sinister increase in mortality.

For all the mass of data which doctors have gathered about the disease, its cause remains a riddle that may take many years to solve. Several pointers have, however, emerged from the mountainous body of facts and figures on which we base our current knowledge. But perhaps the only direct inference we may draw is that no one can yet dogmatize about heart disease; at best he can join a school of thought, and many of these exist.

In the case against coronary artery disease, the major indictment has fallen on fat, and one in particular: cholesterol. This substance invades the arteries and, linked with other fats, causes them to harden and thicken. These fatty deposits on the smooth inner lining of blood vessels attract calcium which helps to form a layer of hard, porridgy material. In the same way that hard water clogs a household pipe, this fatty substance furs up the walls of the arteries; the smooth lining is attacked and blood clots begin to form which block the arteries; or the arterial walls weaken so much that they begin to balloon and finally rupture, causing a massive haemorrhage. Cholesterol has been isolated from clogged and burst arteries and would appear to play some part in atherosclerosis—hardening of the arteries.

Since cholesterol is a fat, doctors turned their attention to the diet as a factor in coronary artery disease. Soon, ample evidence accumulated to support their findings in the laboratory and in the operating theatre. Western countries, with their high-fat diets and their richer foods, suffered much more from coronary disease than Africans or Asiatics who lived on maize, rice, fish and vegetables. Several curious pieces of information seemed to endorse the fat theory. The Japanese, who eat predominantly fish and rice, have a low coronary rate; but those Japanese who emigrate to Hawaii and adopt American eating habits acquire the same susceptibility to heart disease as the U.S. community. Studies carried out among the native and white populations of South Africa underline the dramatic difference between the Bantu, who live on wheat products and have little heart trouble, and the white population with their high-protein diet and the correspondingly high coronary rate.

There would appear good grounds for linking high fat consumption with coronary artery disease, but certain discrepancies have cropped up in the general pattern. How can the statistician reconcile the fact that countries like Denmark, Norway and Holland which eat a great deal of fat have a relatively low coronary incidence, while Scotland, New Zealand and Finland with similar dietary habits lose so many people in their prime to the disease? Nonetheless, the disease does seem to fasten on those countries which eat rich food— possibly too much of it.

Several scientists, notably Dr. Hugh Sinclair of Oxford University, have suggested that some fats may do the arteries more harm than others. This school argues that refining and hardening of fats destroy their essential acids and make it difficult for the body to cope with them. So some authorities advocate eating fats which contain these essential acids, namely corn and some other vegetable oils. By no means all research workers subscribe to this view, since the link between cholesterol and coronary thrombosis has not yet been firmly established. For instance, wartime studies in Britain and Norway showed that, while these countries had to accept a high-fat diet, their incidence of coronary artery disease actually declined. Another curious piece of evidence which seemed to refute the cholesterol theory came from research done during the Korean war. American doctors discovered to their astonishment that young servicemen killed in the fighting had fatty deposits of cholesterol in their major arteries. If cholesterol kills, it must therefore lie latent many years before doing so.

Professor John Yudkin, head of the Department of Nutrition at London University, looked at all the statistics on the relation between dietary fat and coronary thrombosis and concluded that no single factor in the diet affected the incidence of the disease. He did find, however, a remarkable correlation between the increase of heart disease and the numbers of motor cars, radio and TV licences!

Yudkin's finding implies that leisure may play as big a part as any other factor in coronary thrombosis, and this has shown up in hundreds of studies, the incidence of the disease running parallel with the amount of leisure a country enjoys. The heart can withstand any amount of punishment but it would seem that inactivity affects it in two ways: the supply to its coronary arteries decreases and the arteries constrict; secondly, the extra weight which the sedentary person carries round imposes a great strain on the heart arteries.

London Transport made a survey of the effects of heart artery disease on their bus drivers and conductors. The drivers who sat at their work—and perhaps did their job under greater stress—had more coronary disease than the conductors who spent their time running up and down stairs. Exercise, which certainly improves the blood circulation to the heart, also appears to help after a thrombosis by increasing the blood supply in the undamaged part of the organ.

The other factor which has received much attention is stress. The executive seems more likely to succumb to heart seizures than the labourer, and this has been attributed to the pace at which he works and lives and the worry of his job.

The whole picture of coronary disease is slightly blurred round the edges. Many a long, and wrong inference has been drawn from medical statistics, and the pattern of coronary disease is complicated by so many different notions. To the causes which have been mentioned can be added tobacco, for it seems that smoking increases the risk of coronary attacks. It is likely, too, that climate, the type of water, and even the type of soil may play some role in the final balance-sheet of the disease. The patchwork character of the cause and effect in heart trouble means that prevention must necessarily take second place to treatment.

Whatever the cause, coronary thrombosis strikes dramatically, blocking off nourishment to the heart itself and often stopping the organ altogether. However sudden the attack, the disease begins as a slow, insidious siege on the heart arteries; the process takes many years before the blockage makes the patient aware of the crushing, vice-like chest pain, the choking breathlessness, the fever and the nightmare idea of impending dissolution which typify heart seizures.

In its lifetime the heart stands up to tremendous punishment; but nowhere does it behave more impressively than when it meets an assault on its own arteries. These coronary arteries—so-called because they twine like a crown round the heart—play a vital part in the body. Fed by blood from the aorta, they push it at pressure into the two main channels round the heart and into a tracery of fine vessels which thread themselves through the main heart muscle. The heart, working two to three times as hard as the legs of a top sprinter, is the greediest consumer of oxygen and nutrients in the body; other organs can make do with only a quarter of the oxygen transported to them by blood; the heart must consume four-fifths. Nevertheless, in comparison with other organs, the heart comes off poorly in terms of blood supply. Only a tenth of the total amount of blood passing through the body is diverted to feed the heart, while the kidney gets about a quarter. To make up for the relatively low blood supply the heart has become more adept at extracting oxygen and nourishment from its blood.

Paradoxically, its high demands and its very efficiency leave the heart badly off when it faces a crisis. Any decline in blood supply affects it profoundly, and it cannot improve on its already highly-developed thrift. Hence it possesses few built-in safety factors when one of its own arteries fails.

The blocking of a coronary artery does not mean death. Far from it. With a main blood pipe out of action the heart, however crippled, will, in four out of five cases, maintain some sort of function. Its muscle will even grow new tendrils of blood vessels to help supply muscle which has been starved by the blocked artery.

By and large the physician has no answer to heart disease. Angina pectoris he can help, with amyl nitrate, which is broken in its phial and inhaled, or nitroglycerine, in the form of tablets which are sucked. Both these drugs dilate the heart arteries and relieve attacks.

Surgeons have, however, evolved several ways of dealing with angina—from severing the nerves which supply the heart to direct operations on the heart itself.

At the turn of the century, a French physiologist first suggested blocking off the heart nerves to relieve the pain of angina, and, incidentally, to remove the fear which accompanies and intensifies attacks. Seventeen years later, the Rumanian surgeon, Thomas Jonnesco, cut these nerve fibres which lead from the heart into the main nerve pathways along the spine. His patient, a man of 28, said he had complete relief from pain for the next four years. The operation of these sympathetic nerves was followed up by the great surgeon Professor René Leriche, of Strassbourg, who devised methods of excising the nerves, or blocking them with injections of drugs. These operations, still practised, relieve only the pain and do little for the condition which causes it.

Another operation, which had a shorter vogue, was the removal of parts of the thyroid gland which controls the rate at which the body cells burn their energy. By cutting out this gland the heart worked slower and therefore placed less strain on its defective arteries. But the side-effects of thyroid operation deterred even the boldest surgeons and gradually relegated the operation to a footnote in the textbooks.

Though coronary thrombosis presents such problems, surgeons have not given up hope of completely relieving it. The man who has achieved most in the surgical treatment of the damaged heart muscle is Professor Claude Beck, of Cleveland. He first became interested in the diseases which attacked the heart in 1923, when most physicians still had to do their homework at the mention of coronary artery disease. Over the years, Beck pondered how the surgeon might repair the arteries which supplied the heart when they narrowed in angina, or blocked in coronary thrombosis.

In 1932, the idea struck him of channelling blood from other parts of the body into the starved heart. Hundreds of experimental operations had already convinced him of the futility of scraping out furred arteries ; or of trying to repair the arteries themselves.

Blood starvation, he knew, caused the heart to stop. But how and why? He and other observers noticed that the heart often fibrillated wildly before halting completely. The organ never rebelled if it were fully supplied with oxygen; more surprising, Beck proved that a heart deprived completely of oxygen kept its stability. He drew the conclusions that differences of oxygen supply to the muscles which were alive and those which had died caused the fibrillation, threw the heart out of its stride and stopped it. The electrical impulses which kept the heart in rhythm went wild and, as Beck said, the organ electrocuted itself.

We have all heard of these people who die because their hearts literally short-circuit current from pink, healthy muscle to blue, diseased tissue. Beck cited the man who goes out to shovel snow off his path—and drops dead. He had been struck down by a coronary, but Beck contends that he need not have had a bad heart. What happened was this: the un-wonted exercise drove blood into the coronary arteries and this raised the currents through the healthy muscle. But where the blood supply had been arrested or hampered by blockage or thickening of arteries the electrical current remained low. The difference in these electrical impulses was sufficient to short-circuit the heart, send it into fibrillation and stop it.

Increasing the blood flow to the heart would nourish the muscle and stop the blue-and-pink patchwork effect which produced the killing shocks. Beck had also observed during his experimental work that, given a chance, the heart muscle would put out new tendrils to nourish itself with blood. What he had done experimentally could surely be repeated in the operating theatre, Beck told himself, and got busy devising a surgical technique and looking for a patient.

In the mid-thirties it was no light task. And even a deter-mined spirit like Beck saw the dangers of the procedure. How, for example, would the heart react to such major surgery? If the operation succeeded would not the grafted tissue hinder its free movement? It did not seem so in animals; but man may always respond in a different way.

As the Cleveland professor said, "To select a satisfactory case was not without difficulty, and then for the selected patient to give his consent to have an operation performed (an operation that had never been done before on a human being) required something of an heroic spirit."

But such a patient existed and was willing to place his life in Beck's hands. Joseph Krchmar was 48 when his doctor in Chardon, Ohio, referred him to the surgeon. For nine years a vicious pain over his heart and breastbone had plagued him. As a miner, he remembered the minute the pain had seized him while he worked and turned him into a breathless, agonized creature. He stuck at the coal face for another five years before his heart trouble forced him to give up and take a lighter job on a farm; though even there he had bouts of teeth-gritting agony in his chest, heart and down the left arm.

Krchmar was well-developed, but Beck noted the worried expression beneath his beetling brows and dark hair. He told the surgeon that he had just got over a very bad attack ten days before he reported to hospital. When he came into the Lakeside Hospital in Cleveland, he had another spasm which left him breathless, weak and with the slight bluish colour which points to lack of blood oxygen.

Yes, he would have the operation. But could he go to visit his family first. On the eve of the operation Krchmar went home to stay the night—but at midnight he came back to the hospital suffering from still another heart attack. In those days he could hardly be considered a safe candidate for a long, arduous and untried operation.

Beck had sketched out in meticulous detail the way in which he would carry out the task on the 13th of February, 1935. He would rely on light anaesthesia, make a half-moon incision round the heart, take out the ribs and expose the organ.

This he did; then, slitting the pericardium, the moist envelope of the heart, he took a burr and roughened its outer lining so that it would "take" when grafted to the chest muscle. Again he employed the burr to shred off the inside of the pericardium—and this time the heart complained by faltering in its stride and dilating slightly.

Beck and his staff stood back until it had regained its regular beat before they continued with the next part of the operation.

The surgeon had chosen to make his graft from the chest muscle which contained its own arterial supply of blood. Out of this he cut a flap, one end of which he left attached to the chest. The loose end he split into two, and he stitched both flaps to the heart sac. For the final phase of the operation he sewed the graft and the pericardium on to the surface of the heart.

Beck watched his patient carefully during the next months. Krchmar remained in hospital, doing various jobs around the ward for a month or two. The operation seemed to have done him good: gone was his worried frown; and his attacks had disappeared. Seven months later Beck had done another five patients—and his first one had started his farm work again.

In September of that year, the surgeon announced his results to a meeting of the American Surgical Association in Boston. Here, he took the unusual step of mentioning Krchmar by name for his "heroic spirit" in submitting to the operation. "I believe," said Beck, "he has made a contribution to surgery."

Eight years later Krchmar was able to write to his surgeon and tell him he was working twelve hours a day on his farm. "Feeling fine," he wrote, "and able to work hard every day."

By then Beck had done thirty-seven operations and had many such testimonials from patients whose lives he had changed.

The operating mortality ran fairly high as it does with any new and major surgical treatment, but the skill of the team at Cleveland soon reduced the death rate. They expected mistakes at the beginning and realized they were dealing with poor-risk patients. The Beck team had their reward in the improvement of those who were cardiac cripples and who went back to their work.

The surgeon did not rest satisfied with the technique he had devised for Krchmar. He sought means of simplifying the procedure and of boosting the blood supply to the coronary arteries. Toiling long days with experimental animals he worked out modifications of his operation which gave better results. He also took great care in selecting those patients whom the operation would help. Beck does not believe in keeping his patients in the dark. He persuades his patients to give up smoking; he conditions them to adapt themselves to the nursing after their surgery; and he explains the various steps of the operation to them.

The Cleveland professor has improved his technique for providing new blood channels to the heart and, at the same time, reduced the surgery to a surface operation which can be carried out under light general anaesthesia with muscular relaxation. He lays the patient on the right side and approaches the heart through a long incision between the fifth and sixth ribs. Holding the ribs apart with a special retractor, Beck then examines the heart to see if it is enlarged, if the beat is regular and if it shows signs of coronary damage. By probing with the fingers the surgeon can tell if the arteries have blocked or even thickened. By tipping the heart over he can look at the reverse side for arterial damage.

When the heart has been examined the operation begins with the surgeon scraping the surface of the pericardium with special burrs. That done, the heart is rotated to bring up one of its main veins. To redistribute the blood through the heart muscle this vein is partially tied off with silk thread. The surface of the heart muscle is then gently roughened between the branches of the arteries and moistened with a weak acid solution to prepare the organ for its graft. The operation is then completed by sprinkling the surface of the heart with powdered asbestos to create inflammation which will help the muscle to grow new blood vessels. Fat, brought up from the pericardium and its surroundings, is sewn on to the heart muscle and the surgery is completed.

Between the beginning of 1954 and the spring of 1958, at the Mount Sinai and University Hospitals in Cleveland, Beck and his team did this operation on 347 patients. Considering that most of these patients had advanced heart disease—a third were in the terminal stage and many were grave surgical risks—the results proved nothing short of astounding. Only six in every 100 patients died. But Beck achieved the remarkable record of 100 consecutive operations without mortality; in 200 successive cases he had no more than four deaths.

In the hands of a less experienced surgeon the death rate must have been higher. For Beck reported that many of his successful cases "died" on the table and were brought back to life with heart massage and shock treatment. With some patients they toiled as long as sixteen hours to resuscitate their hearts. Perhaps the strangest fact of all, some of these patients woke up after dying and spoke to the surgeons who were working to keep their hearts going. "One patient," said Beck, "between these temporary deaths, stated that she did not like the electric shocks, that she thought they were only for psychiatric patients."

The Cleveland surgeons followed up their cases. Out of the series, 94 in over 100 either had an "excellent" or a "good" rating; the majority had gone back to their regular work. They felt better, much fitter and had less trouble with cold hands and limbs.

Another surgeon attacked the problem of replenishing the heart vessels in a novel manner. Like Beck, Canadian surgeon

Dr. Arthur Vineberg realized that the heart muscle would carry on if nourished with fresh blood in the places where its own arteries had failed. In 1945, Vineberg began experiments at the Department of Surgery, McGill University, to see if he could develop a new blood irrigation system for the dry areas of the heart. The organ, he explained, has a sponge-like network of vessels which are free from furring or blockage and need only to be fed with blood. But most of these blood vessels, according to Vineberg, were buried deep in the thick heart muscles and the surgeon had therefore to devise methods of infiltrating blood into them.

Vineberg's solution was ingenious. He tunnelled deep into the wall of the heart and prepared a bed. He then freed one of the arteries running just inside the chest wall. One end of this artery he tied off; the other he brought to the hole which he had made in the heart wall, and implanted its bleeding end into it. Vineberg reasoned that the bleeding end of this artery would keep pumping blood into the heart vessels until they formed alternative channels of their own. In 1950, Vineberg performed the first of many such operations on patients with coronary artery disease and the results indicated that the procedure helped to abolish the pain and the strain of the condition and increase the life span.

Beck and Vineberg have attracted a good many surgeons to their techniques, although these have by no means gained general acceptance, depending as they do on the skill of the surgeon and his willingness to undertake this type of heart surgery in the face of professional antipathy and even apathy.

Beck, when he reviewed twenty-five years of progress in coronary artery disease before the American Association for Thoracic Surgery in May, 1958, at Boston, took his colleagues to task for their lack of interest in surgical methods of treating coronary disease—what he called "the world's greatest killer".

Beck told the meeting: "There exists a strange complacency

towards this disease. There is no relationship between treatment and death. There is no responsibility for death. This futility has paralysed thinking and has created a belief that to do nothing more than the old routine is to make no mistake. Nowhere in medicine is there such intellectual emptiness as exists in the understanding and treatment of this disease."

Great battalions of doctors are seeking the will-o'-the-wisp clues to coronary disease. The epidemiologist hopes that somewhere in the vast jigsaw of facts and figures about diet and environment he will turn up the vital clue to the prevention or treatment of the disease. The research worker looks hard at the results and wonders if he can equip the physician with the means of reversing or correcting the process of heart disease. The surgeon has to take the direct route and try to repair what is beyond the physician's help. With new techniques of sewing very small vessels together; with further experience of grafting tissue and even replacing it; with the clues which emerge from the patients who have had operations, perhaps the surgeon will win yet another tussle with the heart. If so, he will owe much to Beck and the pioneers who refused to give up.

17

A New Heart in Ten Years?

THE FIFTIES were a golden decade for the heart surgeon —into them he crammed what seemed the work of a century. He owed much to the pure research which flowed from medical laboratories, to the advances in diagnostic methods, to the developments in anaesthesia and antibiotics, and, of course, to the skill of the engineers. Often, though, he had to experiment himself with new approaches to old problems; occasionally he chanced his knife when he ran out of logic or inspiration. However he achieved it, the surgeon of the fifties will attract the attention and admiration of both practitioners and patients as long as medical history lasts.

Now, heart surgery—and other branches of the art—are going through a period of reappraisal, a sort of breath-catching pause to give medicine an opportunity to take stock of what has been accomplished and what remains to do.

A few hardy spirits are ploughing on, hoping for the type of breakthrough which characterized heart surgery in the golden decade; the majority are content to mop up behind the forward leaps which they have made. Men with years of experience of heart-lung machine and hundreds of operations still ask themselves what happens to the circulation when the heart is short-circuited. Hypothermia, too, provokes serious questions from biochemists who are still studying the changes which it must create in the body, in the brain. It may take several years to solve these questions—but even the answers may throw up some fascinating developments.

Several centres in Britain and America are already working on a new type of heart-lung machine. One of the drawbacks to the present machine lies in the system of replenishing the blood oxygen. Donal Effler, who did the first stopped-heart operation, pointed out that the machine might deliver too little oxygen and result in a dangerous rise in blood acid, breathing failure and death; or it might, he contended, over-saturate the blood with oxygen and cause complications, especially in children.

The present machine cannot act as a complete substitute for the heart and lungs. Its pump appears efficient enough, but the oxygenator needs to be improved and brought more into line with the function of the lungs themselves. At Hammersmith, they believe that the future of the machine depends on creating more lifelike artificial lungs. Studies of porous membranes reveal that these would hold blood in circulation while they "breathed" oxygen and gave off carbon dioxide. Several problems still confront the engineer; the blood tends to trap itself between the layers of artificial tissue and form pools which interfere with the oxygen exchange. The designers have also encountered difficulties in diffusing the oxygen through the blood. But they do not appear too pessimistic about surmounting these obstacles.

Such a heart-lung machine would further cut the risks in heart surgery since it would simulate the work of the lungs almost perfectly. The by-pass operation has always proved most difficult with infants, and the introduction of a machine with plastic lungs would make these operations much easier for the surgeon and safer for the patient. The heart-lung apparatus still remains a comparative newcomer to the operating theatre, and the years are likely to bring many more refinements, if not a completely new type of equipment.

The other great surgical boon, hypothermia, may revolutionize heart surgery within very few years. The surgeons who practise profound cooling predict that they can achieve lower temperatures—to within a few degrees of freezing point. If they can achieve this without detriment to the oxygen dependence of the brain and body they can then switch off life for much longer periods than one hour and carry out more intricate surgery on the heart, the brain and other organs.

Hypothermia has inspired research workers to look for some other way of inducing artificial hibernation. Several groups of scientists are looking at substances which may completely stifle the action of the body for several hours. Such chemicals would abolish the need for heart-lung machines and even anaesthetics.

In Toronto, a research team is working on ways of creating artificial hibernation in man with chemical agents. Bigelow, who began the real surgical drive in hypothermia, believes that the answer to artificial hibernation and the whole problem of hypothermia may lie in some hormone which controls the body responses when animals enter their winter sleep. This hormone may come from the hibernating gland of these animals, circulate in the blood and depress the whole response of the body. Bigelow thinks this chemical may endow the animals with unusual resistance to cold and alter the way in which cells burn food and oxygen. As evidence for this hibernating hormone he cites the fact that new-born animals —and possibly premature children—behave like hibernating animals by having a greater tolerance to cold and an unstable heat-regulating mechanism.

If Bigelow's idea proves right, then this hormone might be isolated and used to bring on artificial hibernation in people. The surgeon could operate under cold-sleep conditions and the patient need not wake up until he had recovered fully. Such artificial hibernation would become not only an invaluable asset to the surgeon: the physician, too, could use long-sleep treatment to tide patients over critical illness. Man, who began by borrowing some of the tricks of the hamster and the squirrel, may soon be in the position to teach them something new.

As several surgeons have demonstrated, death can be snubbed not once but several times, regardless of whether it occurs inside or outside the hospital. Heart massage, the pacemaker and shock therapy have all combined to give the good heart a second chance. But so often both the physician and the surgeon have to stand by and watch people die because their heart has worn out and cannot be jogged back into life. The same applies to other organs—artery disease, kidney and liver trouble can kill just as well as the heart, even though the rest of the body stays healthy.

The modern surgeon has moved forward to meet this problem of how to fit spares to the human body, to replace faulty or defunct organs and permit people who would die prematurely to live out a normal span. Already he can envisage the methods; in a few cases he appears to have met with some success and some hundreds of people are walking round with "plastic props" inside them who would have been dead.

Spare-part surgery, as it is called, began with the replacement of arteries. For diseased arteries account for nearly half the deaths in America and Britain each year.

It was Robert Gross and Clarence Crafoord who in the 1940s first began to graft sections of artery into the aorta when they had cut out the narrowed part of the artery. Other surgeons had already shown that arteries could be opened and scraped clean of the fatty debris which threatened to block them. In 1950, French surgeon Jean Kumlin succeeded in making a detour round a blocked artery by grafting another artery above and below the diseased portion. Artery banks began to spring up in hospitals in France, America and Britain to cope with the new techniques, and surgeons worked to improve their skill at stitching together blood vessels which varied in diameter from the aorta, the size of a garden hose-pipe, down to arteries as thick as heavy electric flex.

Before they were grafted into the body, these blood vessels were carefully sterilized by treatment with antibiotics, or by freezing. Storage in vacuum tubes kept them fresh until the surgeon called for them.

Working with human arteries had its disadvantages: the artery banks relied on the post-mortem rooms for their replacements and this involved ethical problems as well as shortages of material; a more fundamental problem was that these grafts did not "take", and within a few weeks the body into which they had been stitched had disowned them. Thirdly, many of the arteries gave as much trouble as those they replaced, since they either had flaws or were diseased. But these borrowed blood vessels did their job. Surgeons noticed that, regardless of whether an artery settled down in its new body, it acted as a form of scaffolding while nature built new tissues round and through it.

However, many surgeons remained dissatisfied with the natural grafts which, besides their other defects, they could not trim to fit the pieces of blocked, clogged or ruptured arteries they excised. They started a search for some material which the body might accept and which would last as long as it might be needed.

In 1952, three American surgeons made the observation which gave spare-part surgery new impetus. Dr. A. B. Voorhees and two colleagues noticed that a single strand of silk which had been placed in the right ventricle of a heart had become coated with blood—and it showed no sign of clotting. They followed up this clue by doing several months of experimental studies with porous plastic cloth which they cut, shaped and inserted into the arteries of animals. They had guessed right; the arterial blood did not leak through the cloth but formed a sheath round it through which the circulation maintained itself. There seemed, too, no reaction by the body against this synthetic material.

The work of Voorhees virtually closed down the artery banks. Who, after all, needed these when you could do much better with plastic shirting material and a sewing machine? Materials like Terylene or Orlon could be cut and sewn in a few minutes to suit the smallest and the largest arteries; they proved easier to suture and raised none of the problems of blood leaks at their junctions which had plagued surgeons working with human grafts. In the early fifties industrial chemists produced a hard, white plastic with the jaw-breaking chemical name, polytetrafluorethylene, known by the trade names Fluon and Teflon. The slipperiest stuff in the world, PTFE also has the big asset of being one of the most inert materials known. Proof against water and acid, PTFE can be cut, moulded and fitted into the body to last a lifetime. With this and Terylene, surgeons can now section large ballooning arteries and replace them; they can by-pass blockages or stiffen weak blood vessels.

The heart machine had solved problems, though it uncovered other snags for the surgeon—first with faulty valves and later with large holes in the inner walls of the heart. Where a valve had merely stuck they could relieve it with the knife; when a hole was small they drew it together with needle and thread. But many valves and holes demanded something more than cutting and suturing.

Where the leaves of valves had been eroded along their edges, or the valve ring itself had stretched, the surgeon could do few repairs with his knife. The two most important heart valves, those on the left side, presented the greatest problem and gave most trouble. If the two-leaved mitral valve became incompetent, this meant that blood, which should have gone out of the left ventricle into the arteries, blew back into the upper chamber and raised the pressure there and even in the lungs. Surgeons like Lillehei in Minneapolis, Kirklin in the Mayo, and Cleland at Hammersmith, did their best with plastic patches. They strutted the edges of the valve; or, if this did not relieve the back pressure, sewed part of the leaves together, narrowing the opening, and patched the remaining section. Lillehei, and another American surgeon, Charles Hufnagel, pioneered the development of complete plastic valves which might be stitched into place between the heart chambers. The first of these valves was simply cut out of plastic, with a narrow opening to allow the blood through and a flap which closed when pressure was applied, to prevent the blood leaking back through the valve. These plastic props corrected some of the reflux of blood from one chamber to another.

Most of the spare-part surgery of the heart has focused on defects in the walls and the aortic valve. It seemed impossible at one stage to achieve anything for patients with aortic valve trouble since this form of "swing-door" lies between the left ventricle and the main blood pipe to all the arteries. When the left ventricle contracts to wring blood into the arteries the pressure on this valve snaps it shut with a sound which the physician can easily hear through a stethoscope. Any weakness in this valve is soon emphasized by the blood pounding against it; and few hearts or bodies stand up for long to any trouble at the main blood outlet. Credit for the first real attempt to correct deformities of the aortic valve must go to Charles Hufnagel who, in 1953, hit on the idea of replacing the whole of the valve with the type of ball valve used in industry. Hufnagel cut away part of the aorta as it swept downward from the heart to the trunk and crimped the valve into the two ends of the blood vessel. Later, he excised larger portions of the aorta and fitted plastic tubing on either side of the large valve. The results encouraged him and a few other surgeons to carry on— only a quarter of the arterial flow ebbed back through the valve. At first, patients went round with the valve clicking inside their chests, but design refinements have made the artificial valves noiseless.

Kolff, of Cleveland, has devised single leaves for diseased aortic valves which a team of surgeons have tried out with success experimentally. But, since the arrival of PTFE, this tough slippery plastic has become the material of choice for man-made valves. The plastic can be cut into a heart shape, with three segments designed like the three leaves of the aortic valve. These segments overlap, so that the blood may be pushed through into the aorta, but the back pressure forces the valve leaves shut. Several other types of valve exist—including one which Hufnagel invented in 1958 which opens and closes with a coiled spring and will last, its designers say, for sixty years.

No surgeon would claim that these artificial props represent the final solution to heart defects. Nature fashioned the heart valves and muscles over millions of years, and the chemist and the engineer cannot hope to duplicate the efficiency of human creation. But this type of biological engineering has come a long way in a few years and has saved thousands of lives with plastic parts for arteries, heart walls and valves. Even now, some surgeons conceive that, if everything else fails, they may be able to give patients a new heart made of plastic and run by electricity.

The man behind this scheme to replace the heart completely is Dr. Willem Kolff, inventor of the artificial kidney and his own type of heart-lung machine. In May, 1960, Kolff and two colleagues from the Cleveland Clinic Foundation, wrote in the *American Heart Journal*: "It is our aim to construct a pump that can replace permanently the irreparably sick human heart." In their report they described how they had built a pump out of plastic parts, and fitted it into an animal to keep it going—without its own heart—for more than five hours!

The Kolff pump works like a dynamo. Current drives a

motor, placed in the centre of the plastic heart, and causes it to swing to and fro on a rocker arm like a pendulum. As the motor swings against one of the outside walls of the "heart" it squeezes blood into the arteries while the space left on the other side fills with blood. The two ventricles of the heart are thus replaced by one large chamber, and instead of pumping in unison they beat consecutively, But Kolff has found, during laboratory and animal experiments, that in this way he can keep enough blood flowing to maintain the circulation. The dynamo, constructed from inert plastic, does not damage the sensitive blood cells to any dangerous degree. The first animal experiment took place on the 26th of June, 1959. Kolff has since designed more elaborate mechanisms which may even be fitted soon in patients.

The surgeons who replace valves and arteries with synthetic materials realize that these can serve as second-best. Human engineering has not yet reached the point where designers can envisage creating a robot heart which will stand in for the masterpiece nature has taken aeons to develop. Even the valves of the heart, with their delicate tissue which will withstand rugged work for a lifetime, look like defying any attempts at imitation for many years. The surgeon would rather, in fact, use human spare parts to replace those which have worn out or suffered injury.

Technically, no problem presents itself in grafting new tissues into the body. Since 1912, when French surgeon Alexis Carrel received the Nobel Prize for transplanting organs from one animal to another, the research surgeon had demonstrated that the kidney, liver, heart and even the head may be grafted from one body to another. Pre-eminent in this field has been the work of Russian surgeon Vladimir Demikhov. In his Moscow laboratories, Professor Demikhov began with experiments to transplant a heart from one animal to another and keep it beating in its new body. It meant opening the chest and sewing together the main arteries and veins from both hearts—a feat which demanded fine surgical dexterity. In 1949, Demikhov was able to report success. The second-hand heart had been coupled in parallel with the old one and was beating in unison with it. For ten days both hearts kept going, then suddenly the animals died. The Russian surgeon carried on perfecting his technique of stitching blood vessels together and watching the reaction of the graft in its new home. In 1956 he performed an incredible surgical *tour de force* by grafting the head of one puppy on to the neck of another puppy. For a week, the surgeon and his staff observed the two-headed animal leading a normal life and seemingly using all its senses with both heads. Demikhov had confirmed what surgeons have known for many years: there are few organs which cannot be transplanted from one body to another with present surgical techniques.

But Demikhov's dogs had one factor in common. Every one of them died. If the new graft did not kill them they killed it. It was the old story of arterial grafts, or almost any other form of human graft—the body rebelled and destroyed them. This incompatibility between a graft and its host makes spare-part surgery impossible at present.

To understand how grafts are rejected, research teams began to look at the way in which the body rigged its defences against other intruders. Vaccination, originated by Edward Jenner in 1796, provided the classical example of the way in which the human system copes with germs. A small dose of cowpox virus will provoke antibodies or defence agents which attack and kill the germs. The germs need not even be alive in order to provoke resistance from the body; some vaccines are put together from virus particles killed in strong chemicals and these—polio vaccine is the best example—produce strong antibody reactions. If the body could immunize itself against virus, it could equally well ward off foreign materials with the same mechanism, the research workers reasoned.

So it turned out. The grafts which plastic surgeons cut from one body and sewed to another sloughed off after two or three weeks; arteries fared no better; and even some inanimate materials aroused foreign-body reactions. There were exceptions. For example, blood may be transfused from one person to another provided the blood groups are matched, though individuals will die if given transfusions from any of the three blood groups other than their own. Corneal grafts can be taken from a person, stored for years, and then transplanted with every hope that they will "take" permanently. The same applies to cartilage.

Outside of these three substances, nothing will survive if lifted from its own body and placed in another. Man, it seemed, was unique biologically. Just as no two fingerprints looked alike under close scrutiny, so no two human beings had the same body chemistry. And the subtleties of each body were enough to wreck the chances of spare-part surgery.

One important exception gave research workers the lead they wanted—identical twins. These twins, born from the same cell, have the same body chemistry and will accept grafts from each other. The scientist began to look more closely at twins, both identical and non-identical, in the human and the animal kingdom. It was an American scientist who first noticed that in some cases non-identical twin calves could acquire tolerance to cells transplanted between them. In 1945, Dr. Ray D. Owen reported his findings and suggested that because they shared a blood circulation before birth these twins had inoculated each other with a transfusion of cells.

This piece of information meant little to anyone except geneticists and made little impact on the scientific world. But one man seized on it and out of it rigged a whole new concept of immunology which gained him and another scientist the

1960 Nobel Prize in medicine. Professor Frank Macfarlane Burnet, Director of the Walter and Eliza Hall Institute for Medical Research in Melbourne, set to work on Owen's discovery and within a few years had published his new theory of how the human body may react to vaccines or viruses and other foreign substances.

In his middle fifties, Burnet had crammed several careers into his working life. A virologist of world reputation, he had helped to isolate and tame the microbe causing psittacosis, the parrot disease which attacks human beings; he had led the postwar research into new strains of influenza virus and vaccines to combat them; and he had drawn attention to various perplexities in the current theories of how people built up immunity to germs. From the early nineteenth century, theorists had wrestled with the puzzle of how the body defended itself against viruses which caused smallpox, flu, polio and the common cold. They had postulated that body cells reacted to certain parts of a virus or other foreign substance and manufactured antibodies corresponding to the substance. As a key fits a particular lock, so the antibody matched the part of the material which had tried to attack the cells. Since protective antibody can be measured only after invasion by a foreign substance, this theory seemed unshakeable.

Burnet, however, asked himself questions which the orthodox theory could not answer. How, for example, can individuals who have suffered isolated attacks of virus disease produce antibodies up to sixty years later? How, in some diseases such as rheumatoid arthritis, can the immune reaction turn and attack the body which it should protect? Owen's observation threw up another conundrum: how do non-identical twins share two different blood groups and defy the universal medical law by accepting skin grafts from each other?

The Australian's solution to these riddles created in effect a completely new theory of immunology which inspired other laboratory teams to test it. Burnet contradicted the notion that antibodies arose out of a form of collision between the invading virus and the cell. The body, he proposed, had a complete alphabet of antibodies in its cells and could manufacture any protective substance when it ever had any need to do so. This set of instructions for making antibodies was contained in the cells along with the hereditary information carried by the genes, the minute particles which decide the characteristics of each individual. Burnet suggested that the body "learned" its alphabet in the early months of its formation through spontaneous changes in the basic properties of the cells.

Burnet's theory appealed to a great many doctors and scientists. Not long after he had outlined the selective theory of immunology, doctors began to pick up instances of non-identical twin children who might accept grafts from each other. Three pairs were discovered who had shared a common blood supply in the womb, and one of these pairs proved that cross-grafting would work. Would it, however, succeed when tried experimentally on animals who were not twins?

This problem occupied three British scientists who had followed the work done by the Australian. They decided to find out if they could play a "genetic trick" on mice by mixing up the cells of one strain with those of another before birth and then attempting to graft between the strains.

Dr. Peter Medawar, Professor of Zoology at London University, and his colleagues, Dr. Leslie Brent and Dr. Rupert Billingham, were engaged on another problem when they decided to follow up Burnet's work. An agriculturalist had approached them to see if they could evolve a sound method of distinguishing between identical and non-identical calves. Medaware reasoned that grafts would take between the identical animals and fail in the others. He proved himself wrong; in fact, nine out of every ten grafts survived transplantation in the non-identical calves. The animals had obviously acquired a tolerance to cells from their twins while they shared a common blood supply before birth. Medawar then planned the experiment which brought him the Nobel Prize, with Burnet. He and his collaborators chose two different strains of brown and white mice. They waited until several mice of the white strain were pregnant and then took spleen cells from the other strain. They operated on the first strain of mice, exposed their babies in the womb and injected the foreign blood cells into them. If they were right in their assumption these foreign cells would confer protection on the baby mice to grafts from the donor strain. After the mice were born they cut skin—the most difficult tissue to graft permanently—from the donor mice and transplanted it in the newborn mice. The brown grafts, which would ordinarily have sloughed off within a few weeks, grew and flourished on the backs of the white mice. Here, the British research team had demonstrated that spare-part surgery was possible—an academic proof, certainly, but one which gave hope to a great many men in laboratories and operating theatre. No one could envisage such a technique as Medawar used ever being applied in practice, but it began a hunt for other methods of damping down the rebellion of the body cells to foreign intrusion.

One of the most important clues came in a tragic way from a science which was advancing just as fast as heart surgery—atomic energy. Nuclear radiations had helped the doctor, first in diagnosis and later in treatment, for a half century, but it was only on the 2nd of December, 1942, that the Italian, Dr. Enrico Fermi, built and operated the first "pile" in Chicago. Since the end of the war atom furnaces have sprung up all over the world, to create electrical power, to make radio-isotopes for medicine, industry and agriculture and to do research. One of these research furnaces was built at Vinca, near the Yugoslav capital, Belgrade, to teach scientists how to construct larger reactors. From this atom research station emerged

the story which set physicians and surgeons talking and thinking throughout the world.

The reactor was small; its enriched uranium fuel kept in
check by heavy water and control rods of special metals. It
had run for some time at the Boris Kidric Institute, before five
men and a woman started a new experiment on the 15th of
October, 1958. Everything seemed to be working properly
and the six scientists were moving round the face of the pile
carrying out their measurements when one of them spotted
something which stopped all of them in their tracks—his film
badge had gone black! To blacken the sensitive emulsion on
the safety film he and the others must have stood in a steady
stream of radiation; the reactor must have run away, melted its
uranium fuel rods and released radio-active particles into the
containment building. Hurriedly, they dropped what they
were doing and got out. As they feared, radio-activity had
escaped. A quick check on their film badges revealed they had
possibly received somewhere between 500 and 1,000 units of
radio-activity—the same dose which had killed people in the
bombed cities of Hiroshima and Nagasaki.

The Yugoslav authorities decided immediately to fly the six
scientists to Paris and a special plane, with protective shielding
for the crew, took off within a few hours of the accident.
None of the young scientists looked ill; they felt normal. But
the health safety authorities at Vinca knew that within a few
weeks they might die from radiation sickness; indeed few
atom doctors who looked at the film badges would have given
them a chance of surviving. The Curie Foundation in Paris had
a modern hospital with 50 years of experience of radiation
medicine behind it. Alerted by the Yugoslav Embassy it stood
by to take in the scientists.

At Orly Airport, the arrival of the scientists caused a temporary scare, until French doctors reassured the public that no
danger from radio-activity existed. At the Curie Hospital

separate rooms had been prepared on the second floor and nurses prepared transfusion equipment in case the blood cells had been so badly damaged that they had to be replaced. Dr. Henri Jammet, Director of the health protection services of the French Atomic Energy Commissariat, was called in to handle the treatment. He and other doctors at the Curie Hospital knew from previous experience what happened in these radiation injuries; large doses destroyed the bone marrow which manu-factures the blood cells. The dose these patients had received might have killed all the bone marrow cells. They just hoped not.

For three weeks they watched the Yugoslavs. One of them, 24-year-old Zivato Vranic, a nuclear engineer who had been working nearest the reactor, showed the first signs of severe radiation injury. Then the others, with one exception, began to suffer from weakness, loss of appetite, falling hair and eye trouble. Their blood counts revealed that they were low in red and white cells.

Dr. Jammet had requested the help of two other specialists in this type of illness—Dr. Jean Bernard and Dr. Georges Mathé. To the three doctors it became obvious that without treatment they could only hope to save one of the scientists. But what treatment? The doctors reasoned that transfusions would help but not overcome their problem, since the bone marrow would not replace blood cells. If only they could give a transfusion of bone marrow which might then take over the creation of new blood cells? No one had ever done it, for the same reason that no one had ever succeeded in transplanting an organ—the body would merely reject the intruding sub-stance. But here, surely, there was a difference. The radiation had destroyed the bone marrow cells. Might it not also have eradicated the antibodies which would normally refuse grafts? From the Curie Hospital, a call went out for volunteers to give bone marrow to the Yugoslav scientists. The people who had read of the case and of the death of Vranic in the middle of

November came in dozens to the hospital. Jammet, Bernard and Mathé picked those with matching blood groups and drew off bone marrow through holes drilled in their ribs and hips. This they fed through tubes into the blood stream of the four patients who had radiation damage. They watched it replenish the depleted marrow in the bones and then create fresh blood; and with repeated grafts, they saw their patients slowly recover until, at the end of April, the four men and their woman colleague left Paris for Yugoslavia.

The Vinca case inspired Bernard and Mathé to try the same technique on patients in the final phase of leukaemia. With radiation they killed off the bone marrow which was making leukaemic cells and then grafted new marrow into patients to prolong their lives. But Vinca had also provided a vital impetus for research doctors who were seeking ways of adapting the body to live with their grafts. If the body responses could be stifled to allow the graft time to take in the case of bone marrow it might work with other transplants.

Several surgeons had, in fact, anticipated many of the results which emerged from the Vinca accident and had already begun experiments with radiation, aiming to damp down the fierce reaction of the body to any foreign invasion. Foremost among these investigators was a young Scots surgeon in the Postgraduate Medical School at Hammersmith Hospital—William J. Dempster. Since 1949 this experimental surgeon had been studying the mechanism which caused grafts to melt and slough off within a few weeks of being transferred from one human being to another. Like Burnet and Medawar, he believed the rejection of these grafts to be caused by antibodies produced by the human cell. Since no two individuals are genetically alike—identical twins excepted—the surgeon had to tackle each case as he met it; had to attempt to break down this uniqueness which stamps everyone subtly but surely in a different chemical mould.

Dempster first proved that the body did build defences against foreign tissue. Taking skin from one animal he grafted it on to another animal, knowing that within weeks it would die. Then he tried again, using the same two animals. The second time the skin perished much faster. Therefore, Dempster deduced, the animal receiving the skin had acquired the same sort of immunity against the cells of the donor animal that people develop against disease after they have been vaccinated. It had learned to spot the intruding and offending cells much more quickly at second sight. But the revulsion of a body against grafts appeared to have a more basic reason—one as fundamental as the difference in every set of fingerprints— a genetic reason. Thus, the question became: how can we trick the body into accepting grafts from a stranger? It was a poser which left both the immunologist and the geneticist groping and bewildered. But surgeons cannot wait until the theorist has finished and the text-books of immunology and genetics have been re-written. They began to look for their own methods.

The academic and experimental technique of Medawar seemed, for the time being, a blind alley to surgeons who were seeking a practical method of making grafts stick permanently. To inoculate mice before birth with cells from another strain fell quite easily within laboratory techniques; to appropriate the technique to human beings presented insurmountable obstacles. So Dempster and his colleagues at the Postgraduate Medical School took a different tack. They realized that X-rays inhibited the growth of tumours and might therefore interrupt the mechanism of the human cells long enough for a new graft to settle in another body. In 1949, they decided to try to quell the normal reaction to grafts with massive doses of X-rays.

So far as the transplantation of skin went, the research surgeons were right. Animals which had received large doses of X-rays accepted grafts for much longer than those which had not been treated. Would it work with other organs? One part of the body lent itself to such experiments: the kidney. One of the most delicate organs in the body, it specializes in disposal of wastes in the blood stream and regulates the balance of chemicals and nutrient in the blood. The kidneys, easily damaged or diseased, offer the surgeon unique opportunity to carry out transplantation, since the human body survives readily on one kidney. In 1954, Dr. John P. Merrill, Dr. J. Hartwell Harrison and Dr. Joseph E. Murray, of the Peter Bent Brigham Hospital in Boston, took a kidney from one young man and grafted it into his twin brother who survived to prove that kidney grafting was possible.

But when Dempster and his colleagues came to apply their radiation technique to kidney grafting between different genetic types, the results disappointed them. The kidney seemed to behave quite unlike skin, for the body threw it off almost as though the surgeons had used no radiation treatment. Experiments convinced Dempster that the kidney itself was rebelling against the body in some way which the Burnet-Medawar theory did not explain. The Hammersmith surgeon proved that the organ played some part in its own rejection by bombarding it with X-rays when it showed signs of dying. The transplanted kidney then settled down in its new human environment.

Both French and British surgeons have applied the radiation technique in practice. Two French groups have reported success in transplanting kidneys between non-identical twins and between a sister and a brother. At Hammersmith, Dempster's group have performed several operations on people who are quite unrelated genetically. In at least one case, the new graft established itself and has functioned normally in the body. But the surgeons are still appraising their results.

The work at Hammersmith and in France has, however, made it clear that Burnet and Medawar have outlined only part of the story of how people react to foreign substances.

Much experimental work remains for the geneticist, the immunologist and the surgeon before he can borrow a part from
one person and use it to prolong the life of someone else. Many
surgeons are nonetheless optimistic about the future of spare-
part surgery, and Dempster has said that when kidney transplantation has become routine the surgeon may turn to the
heart and solve the problems of replacing a worn-out heart
with a better one. The Hammersmith surgeon believes this
can be achieved within ten years.

From its desperate beginnings at the end of the last century,
heart surgery has emerged as the marriage of the highly refined
art of the surgeon with the strict scientific discipline of a dozen
branches of medical science. Every day brings some new idea,
another piece of information from the laboratory, perhaps a
striking advance in operating technique, or a daring inspiration
of the surgeon. Men like Rehn and Souttar, compelled by their
wish to help dying patients, and their vision of what might be
accomplished in heart surgery, persuaded their colleagues to
look again at the heart. From their example, and the work of
the Sauerbruchs, the Blalocks and the Brocks grew the fan-
tastic feats of modern cardiac surgery. Today, the young
surgeon thinks little of taking over the heart and lungs of a
patient, knows that he can arrest the heart if necessary, realizes
that he can even snuff out life and restore it again. He has
stripped the heart of its awe, without ceasing to respect it; he
has converted the miracles of his elders into the routine and the
commonplace. But still there are the pioneers who are toiling
to achieve full mastery over the heart and the ultimate goal of
replacement surgery. Disease has a Chinese Box aspect, and
the surgeon is aware that as he attains one anatomical frontier
another beckons him onward. He knows that, while he dares
something which no one has done before, he has to make life-
and-death decisions and take the risks which go with them.

Index

About the Author

After spending what he describes as "a particularly anecdoteless childhood" in Ayrshire County, Scotland, where he was born, **Hugh McLeave** attended Glasgow University and received a Master of Arts degree in 1949. Having discovered that he had a flair for writing, he set out on a career in journalism. Since then, he has spent nine of his fourteen years in Fleet Street working as scientific and medical correspondent for the *News Chronicle* and the London *Daily Mail*. His work has taken him all over the world—to India and Burma during World War II, to Russia and Bulgaria after the war, and to Christmas Island in the Pacific to observe the second British H-bomb test in 1957.

At present, Mr. McLeave resides in London with his wife. He is the author of two previous books, as well as numerous magazine articles.